LIGHTNESS OF BODY AND MIND

LIGHTNESS OF BODY AND MIND

A Radical Approach to Weight and Wellness

Sarah Hays Coomer

ROWMAN & LITTLEFIELD
Lanham • Boulder • New York • London

Published by Rowman & Littlefield
A wholly owned subsidiary of The Rowman & Littlefield Publishing Group,
Inc.
4501 Forbes Boulevard, Suite 200, Lanham, Maryland 20706
www.rowman.com

Unit A, Whitacre Mews, 26-34 Stannary Street, London SE11 4AB

British Library Cataloguing in Publication Information Available

Library of Congress Cataloging-in-Publication Data

Names: Hays Coomer, Sarah
Title: Lightness of body and mind : A radical approach to weight and wellness / by Sarah Hays
    Coomer.
Description: Lanham, MD: Rowman & Littlefield, 2016 | Includes bibliographical references and
    index.
Identifiers: LCCN 2015039178 | ISBN 9781442255081 (cloth : alkaline paper) | ISBN
    9781442255098 (electronic)
Subjects: LCSH: Weight loss--Psychological aspects--Popular works. | Food habits--Psychological
    aspects--Popular works.
Classification: LCC RM222.2 .H324 2016 | DDC 613.2--dc23 LC record available at http://
    lccn.loc.gov/2015039178

♾ ™ The paper used in this publication meets the minimum requirements of
American National Standard for Information Sciences Permanence of Paper
for Printed Library Materials, ANSI/NISO Z39.48-1992.

Printed in the United States of America

For Sky

CONTENTS

AUTHOR'S NOTE

The names and identifying details of friends and clients described in this book by first name only have been changed to protect their privacy. Those mentioned by first and last name have consented to the use of their real names, thereby agreeing to be part of this madness. The events described are as accurate as memory allows. I can't guarantee perfection in the far reaches of my mind, but I can guarantee that I have done everything in my power to bring these stories to life in the most unvarnished, truthful way possible. I offer them to you as a testament to what can be achieved when candor, determination, and foolishness prevail.

Part I

Making the Choice

How we spend our days is, of course, how we spend our lives.
—Annie Dillard, *The Writing Life*, 1989

I

LIGHTNESS

Like Wall-E, the Pixar robot who roams a vast landscape beset with rubbish, I find myself lately climbing a mountain of half-read weight-loss books and discarded food containers, raising a white flag and calling for a cease-fire.

I'm a personal trainer and health coach, but I have to confess that I cringe a bit at the associations that conjures. To be clear: CrossFit makes me wince, and you will never, ever find me training for a marathon. If an activity breaks my body in any way, if it doesn't support my well-being, I want no part of it.

What I want—and what my clients want—is unbridled, pain-free, kinetic, renewable wellness. And pulverizing our bodies doesn't get us there.

I've been a trainer for twelve years. During much of that time and for more years than I would like to admit, I was at war with my body and losing the battle. I carried around an extra twenty pounds, claiming they proved my commitment to quality of life over superficial concerns, but that was a lie. The extra weight wasn't the result of eating joyfully with people I loved. It was the result of eating too much for the wrong reasons, mostly alone and at night. Food made me feel calm, so I dove in after dark and spent the following twenty-four hours beating myself up over it, before doing it again, and feeling at peace again for a few delicious moments.

The weight felt heavy on my frame, but I couldn't get it off no matter how many lunges or push-ups I did. It was infuriating. I was a trainer for God's sake! I should be able to do this!

Every day I picked through an avalanche of quick fix promises that poured through my inbox and popped up at the fringes of my web browser. I sifted through research to uncover bits of helpful, new information that occasionally arose amid the wasteland of false leads and passed those tips along to my clients as they struggled with their own roadblocks right alongside me.

As a trainer, I was capable of beating back the fraud, but as a human being, I ached for every high-flying promise to be true—effortless and effective, once and for all. My clients, friends, and I were all in search of the same thing. We wanted a final solution, and we were willing to do whatever it took. Follow this diet; do this workout. It will *definitely* work this time.

But, inevitably, the diet was impossible, and I hated the workout—or the workout was okay but the diet made my armpits stink. Whatever. I couldn't stay motivated to stick with it. I understood each plan in theory. Excellent plan! But no. Not happening.

Finally, I realized that the way we were pursuing weight loss was blindly, spectacularly bass-ackward.

No matter how hard we tried, no matter how much money we spent, how little we ate, or how many pounding workouts we completed, we failed to lose weight and keep it off because we were attempting to dominate our bodies, choking them off instead of bringing them to life.

You can't put a vice on your hunger, and you can't wrestle control of your mind to shrink your body. It doesn't work. Weight loss is unsustainable if it comes at the cost of living well. Boredom and frustration don't breed contentment no matter how skinny you manage to get, and rigid, arbitrary weight loss techniques are a steaming, stinking, giant pile of no-fun.

"Skinny" isn't what we're really yearning for anyway. We're yearning for peace in our own skin under easy, unbothered minds—and that kind of peace won't ever be achieved by depriving ourselves of everything we love while performing mind-numbing exercises in our not-so-spare time.

The concept that wellness or lasting weight loss can emerge from blunt force effort is a myth. It's a fantasy we slide into like a warm bath. We jump in with both feet—the best in us wanting to believe we can do it if we just try hard enough. We muscle our way through frustrating diets and workouts, but the whole pursuit turns out to be a pain in the ass. So we quit. With every failure, our confidence takes a hit, and the next attempt is weakened before it even begins.

Limitation and restriction will never inspire you to awaken your body. They will never allow for an uncomplicated relationship with food. They blunt your spirit, deplete your drive, and leave you continually wondering why you have such a hard time following through—but, under those circumstances, failure makes perfect sense.

After years of useless, unproductive deprivation, our bodies are in full-blown rebellion, hanging on for dear life to every moment of relaxation and grasping at every opportunity for yummy, surreptitious satisfaction. The diets and fitness routines most of us are pursuing have no relationship to the reality of our lives or the passions that move us. So, of course, they fail.

It's a bold and scary thing to let go of traditional mechanisms we've put in place to keep excess weight at bay, but if they don't work, what exactly are we doing? Why do we continue to pummel our bodies into submission when we would get so much further by simply taking better care of them?

When you imagine losing weight, what you're truly aching for is a different sensation of being in your body, an expansive one, breathing and moving lighter and easier than you do now. The ultimate goal isn't weight loss; it's liberation. *Freedom* is what you're after, freedom from discomfort—and the only way to achieve that is by prioritizing vitality and resilience over weight loss.

That straightforward shift brings a glorious, unexpected, and radical release. I've seen it in my own body and in my clients, ranging from one hundred to four hundred pounds. When life is no longer lived in a constant state of vigilance, weighed down by wretched, unattainable rules and regulations, the weight can come off as a welcome side effect—slow, steady, and easy. Strength becomes the new ideal, and weight loss an afterthought.

Instead of restricting foods we love, we should be *supplementing* them with plates piled high with whole, real food, cooked in real oils and spices. Instead of cramming our bodies into dark rooms full of exercise equipment, we should be out exploring; in search of whatever activity we can find to love.

The prize in the end isn't weight loss. The prize is the end of the fixation—authentic wellness that arises out of a lifestyle you genuinely enjoy.

Strength and clarity are what we're actually after, and once we go looking for those, it's a different game altogether.

Instead of trying to dodge doughnut joints on the way home from work, what if the doughnuts breezed past you, irrelevant and inert, because you actually *didn't want them*? What if, on the way home, you were busy looking forward to a dinner that would taste and feel good, so good that deep-fried dough passed through the car window and swallowed in hurried bites at a stoplight didn't sound particularly enticing? What if they sounded more like a sugar rush, a dull headache, a night of uncontrollable cravings, and a heavy morning? How much easier would it be to turn down sugary snacks if the mere thought of them meant *dis*comfort instead of comfort?

We're so busy telling ourselves *not* to eat all the time that eating as much as we want is a victory. And who doesn't want a sweet, molten victory? We're so accustomed to forcing ourselves to exercise that sitting on the couch feels like glorious rebellion. Our inner-adolescents come swinging from the rafters, howling that we will not be tamed. "Take your exercise and shove it, fitness freaks!" Might as well curl up right there with Netflix, a fork, and a coffee cake. Settle in for another night of "me time."

But eventually the heaviness gets too depressing. So we sign up for boot camp; twist our knees; and ache from top to bottom as we curse the rolls on our bellies and declare the entire pursuit of wellness impossible.

Instead of following a generic plan to lose weight in the short term, what if you built a self-directed, unshakable infrastructure to support your health and a body weight that will work for you *for the rest of your life*?

Resuscitate your body and provoke your mind. Make consummate peace with your own flesh, and follow your desires where they naturally lead until you're so distracted by what you love that you have absolutely no reason to eat for no reason. That is the work of this book.

When you step back long enough to let your body lead the way, to figure out what feels right and what feels decidedly wrong, the slander in your head is quieted; and when condemnation and guilt aren't invited to the party, there's no need to medicate anxiety with food. You're free to eat for pleasure and liberated to engage in the stuff of your life— work, love, and creativity—disentangled from the blood-sucking self-derision that currently reduces your brain space by half.

Imagine waking up in the morning in a body that feels light and strong, that moves through the day without twisting itself into contorted positions to disguise its objectionable parts. Imagine what it would be like to raise a glass with friends and sit down to dinner to quench your hunger without a passing thought of what *not* to eat or how much is too much?

Guilt-free indulgence embedded in a life of steady wellness: the paradigm shift is there.

Our prehistoric brains are built to keep us fed and happy. Food equals contentment whether we like it or not, and denying ourselves that pleasure has made us obsessed. That obsession has caught us in a cycle of craving and devouring. We've lost track of the difference between satisfied and overstuffed. In case you hadn't noticed, it doesn't feel good to eat an entire pizza alone in one sitting—but damn if I haven't done it more times than I can count. We're heavier than we want to be because we have lost track of what it means to feel "good."

Twenty pounds isn't the goal. Health. Equanimity. Vitality. Carelessness. Those should be the objects of our obsession, not weight loss. As the fixation subsides, any weight that doesn't feel necessary anymore can come off because you're nurturing your body with what it needs—which sometimes means a salad at lunch and sometimes means queso with your margarita. When you're doing the best you can, when no particular food is evil and your body is worthy of appreciation (in spite of whatever imperfections you might perceive), you're free to make healthier choices because *it feels better* to treat yourself that way, not because you're supposed to do this or that to drop weight. I've seen the results in my clients and in myself. You don't need a diet; you need an overhaul of your aspirations.

To begin, ask yourself one, simple question: "What kind of old lady do I want to be?" Or if you're a guy, "What kind of old man?" Where do you want to end up?

This isn't about visualization. It's an honest assessment of what you would like your life to look like in the distant future. Whether or not you're on track for that future is something you can worry about later. For now, just think about what you'd like to have happen.

For myself, I hold an image of a seventy-year-old woman, standing on a cliff in Malibu, painting a picture of the ocean on an easel with a large, feckless paintbrush. She is strong and weathered, with long, unbridled, white-gray hair, wearing dark blue, boy-cut jeans and a loose, white linen, button-up blouse blowing in the breeze. And dogs, she has three or four dogs frolicking about.

True confession: I may or may not have acquired that image from an estrogen-replacement commercial. I'm actually not sure, but whatever, it works for me. Though I've never painted a canvas in my life, that's the energy of who I want to be and the kind of life I want to live in old age, so the question becomes, "How do I get from here to there?"

Find that core ambition and figure out how to bring it to life in your body *sooner than later*. Whoever your ideal, old lady may be, take the journey backward, and every decision you make in daily life will be informed by that aim. By placing her in the distant future, you remove the temptation to judge the present and create plenty of space to strut, careen, and ease your way from here to there.

Everything you do eventually takes hold in your body. Over time, small, daily rituals shape you. Nobody strives to end up immobile and full of regret. Assuming you're not facing a debilitating medical condition, immobility in old age is most often the result of underutilizing your body. It happens by wasting nights that turn into years fretting over the fact that you have a less-than-perfect body (which we all do) and turning to food to make yourself feel better in the meantime. Those nights are so much better spent *doing things you like to do*, instead of trying to control your body or giving up on it entirely.

Waking up in the morning and comparing the way you *want* to be now to the way you *are* now cuts you off at the knees. If the goal and present reality don't match, nothing about that is going to change before sundown when the next temptation arises. The comparison breeds frustration—so you eat. The following day you reach for a diet plan or exercise routine, but whether or not you manage to lose a few pounds, the obsession with losing weight remains one of the formative forces in your life. Food and exercise continue to be your adversaries, and the battle persists as your days stack up, building a world-class tower of never quite good enough—or thin enough. Are you bored of that battle yet? I know I am.

When you address the problem by banning food and forcing exercise, you're only feeding the dysfunction and perpetuating the cycle. To unseat the habits and weight that are bringing you down, don't deprive yourself; don't run your body into the ground. Flip the quest on its head, and go in search of the things that turn you on, that feed your body. Root out the fixation with being fitter *right now* because, if you're not there yet, spending precious energy beating yourself up about that fact is pure, unmitigated sabotage. You have no option but to start from where you are. The most productive, powerful thing you can do is fill your life, ember by ember, with fire that will blaze your body into the form you imagine.

Shape your life in service of that weathered, old woman. Let her have her old age in a body and mind at peace by putting your energy into creating a series of days that will allow her to come to be. Go in search of what makes you feel alive.

When you loosen your grip and shift your focus to building *in* the good rather than defeating the bad, you'll be astonished what else begins to shift. Without dieting, without regimenting your days or minimizing your hunger, your body will change out from under you. It will settle in, on its own, to a new circumference, without deprivation or manipulation.

And one day, if you keep eating a little better and moving a little more, maybe you'll walk into a dressing room with a stack of jeans, the size you always buy. You'll try them on, and every pair will turn out to be beautifully, butt-saggingly baggy.

When this happens, you will barely be able to breathe, not because of how you look but because this new body will come free of strings attached: no strict diet to adhere to, no punishing exercise regimen to follow. You'll be wildly, spectacularly free of body baggage, and—no matter your weight—your only objective will be to maintain your balance and keep feeding the fire.

A few years ago, I found myself standing in a dressing room just like that, verging on tears, hardly able to recognize myself: body and mind. In the previous year, I developed a disciplined practice of focusing exclusively on well-being over weight loss. Food and exercise became allies, and there was no weight-related goal in sight. The number on the scale was in freefall, dipping below what I ever dreamed possible. My body was in search—on its own—of a new resting place, and I had no idea where it would land.

For the first time in my life, I was inhabiting a body that could perceive which kind of sustenance and effort felt right—in the truest sense—and which didn't. And my mind was allowing that transformation to happen without its customary killjoy meddling. I was nourished and satisfied, healthy and strong.

At the age of sixteen, I began digging a ditch to nowhere with my bare hands in a tireless effort to strip my body of its natural resources and shield myself from the temptations of a life exposed. It took me much too long to figure out that I was actually burying myself in heavy mud as handfuls of debris cascaded back to their original resting places, bringing with them mounds of rubbish picked up at the surface. I misused years of my life in that pursuit.

I could easily have continued digging for decades to come, deeper in the trench and farther from sunlight. But, when I became a trainer and witnessed, up close, my clients, friends, and their daughters and sons in combat with their own bodies, I realized that instead of digging in, we needed to pull ourselves up and out and reach skyward, fully exposed to the elements: the earth, sun, water, and air that give us life. Without those people, their tenacity and surefooted willingness to share their struggles with me, I would never have found my way out. Their stories are included in this book as guideposts to usher us through—or warn us off.

The body I now live in is miraculous to me. It's not muscle-bound or unusually thin, just on the fit side of average, but I am at rest in my skin for the first time in my life. I've got many years between now and the blustery afternoon when my old lady climbs up to the cliff over Malibu with her dogs at her heels, but I have every intention of spending as much of that time as possible immersed in her free, unfettered mindset and her body, strong and lawless.

In the meantime, I have hiked to the top of this particular trash heap to wave my tattered flag in an attempt to get you to put down your weapons. It *is* possible to work toward a healthier body while maintaining your sanity, but to do that, you have to engage in a different kind of warfare. Put down your weapons, and walk out of the theater of war. Go after what you love instead of trying to erase what you hate. Start walking, and keep right on going.

You, too, have a lot of time between now and the realization of your older self. To get from here to there and waste as little time as possible feeling crappy, a choice has to be made about what you want—and actions have to follow. This book is about how to make that choice and what to do afterward to construct a body and mind that you have no intention of giving up because they both feel way too good, just as they are.

There's only one requirement for success. There is one fundamental conviction you *must* bring to the table. You need to know, as sure as the air you breathe, that you do not intend to lie on your deathbed knowing that you spent your entire life despising your own body.

You have to know for a fact that you're not going down like that.

Dance with your demons all you want. In fact, in the pages that follow, you will be asked to know them intimately. They will be some of your most valuable teachers, but with every passing waltz, with every old, familiar rhythm, you will begin to know their trickery; learn the dance; and take the lead. Once in motion, you'll be increasingly drawn to freedom and curious about what it might be like for the space around you to feel different, for your clothes to hover just a little, fluttering over the surface of your skin and giving you room to breathe.

Heavy condemnation of an already heavy body makes no sense. As a trainer and human being, I am seeking a cataclysmic overthrow of the way we're pursuing health and weight loss; a complete rejection of counting, measuring, and boot-camping. Instead, wiggle, wriggle, stretch, bounce, roll, crawl, or otherwise burn your way to a life where the things you love matter a whole lot more than a tired, boring, decades old fixation on getting thin. Being thin is useless if it isn't accompanied by fulfillment. Rewiring the way we go after wellness needs to come first so that any physical changes, weight loss or other-wise, materialize out of a life well lived, emerging unforced and uncon-strained.

If you don't feel quite right, there are activities and foods in the world that you might actually enjoy that can make you feel much, much better. It's just a matter of figuring out what they are. Do not be afraid. There will be cocktails along the way—and carelessness and freedom and openhearted, reckless misadventures to keep you entertained.

Lightness is the point, after all, lightness of body and mind.

Author's Note: I have included a "Toolbox" at the end of each chapter to help you nail down specific action steps. Also, I encourage you to purchase or create a journal, which can be a useful, central location to help you track the steps you're taking and gather your thoughts as you work through the book. But think of both the toolboxes and the journal as utilities, not touchy-feely obligations. They are resources for insight and record-keeping; that's all. Tips on how to use them will follow at the end of each chapter. I like to put pen to paper, but if you prefer to keep track on your phone or computer, do what works for you. Or ignore the toolboxes altogether if you're more of a vibe-y, feel-your-way-through-it sort of a person. Everybody is different. Use these tools in whatever ways you wish.

TOOLBOX

What does your old person's life look and feel like?

Give some serious thought to your old self. Who are you? Where are you? And who are you with? Are you working or retired? What do you do with your free time? How does your body feel as you move through your old person day? What are you wearing?

Make it as specific as you can. Write it down in your journal or on sticky notes on the wall. Create a Pinterest board or an Instagram account for your crazy, lovely old person. Make a playlist of her favorite tunes. Make it concrete. Spend some time bringing your old lady and her surroundings and habits to life.

Find one thing your old self does that you can do too.

Does she keep flowers in her kitchen? Is her home pristine or charm-ingly disheveled? Does she stretch every night before bed? Does she doodle on a note pad while she drinks her coffee? Does she go to the farmer's market on Saturdays? Small, steady routines. Try one, and see if it's a helpful addition to your world.

2

THIRST

After finally losing the weight I pursued for so many years, I stepped out of my front door one night onto the sidewalk under streetlights, braless in a cotton tank top and yoga pants. Thick, southern, summer air wrapped around me, massaging my skin as I walked. Headlights flashed as cars passed outside my purview. I had nothing in my hands: nothing to hang on to, nothing to fear letting go of. Music played on shuffle as I crossed the street with my arms outstretched, reaching as far as my fingertips could take me. They tingled.

This body was new. I had no context for what it meant to walk down the street in a body that felt right. My days up until now were filled with sucking in and assembling disguises from an ill-fitting closet. I realized I could not have imagined—even a few months earlier—what it might be like to step out for this stroll, enveloped in darkness, open and upright. I had achieved my own personal version of featherweight. I was free of the weight and, even better, the psychological disquiet that held my body prisoner for decades.

As I walked, I tried to wrap my head around how to communicate this extraordinary, wordless liberation to my clients in a way that could be useful rather than taunting or frustratingly out of reach; how to help them strive for strength rather than trying to dismantle themselves.

Self-help experts would have us "act as if we already are" thinner or more confident, but I've always found this sort of instruction confusing.

It feels like a lie. Pretending to be happy or healthy when I know I'm not only breaks my heart a little deeper. It brings the cavernous gap between what I am and what I want to be into sharp relief. To their credit, what these people actually mean, when they tell you to pretend, is that if you *act* like you're thin, you'll lose weight—because you'll eat less and exercise more; because you'll be doing all the things thin people do; because you'll be acting like you're thin. This kind of circular thinking makes me want to sit down with a cocktail and a bowl of peanuts to get my bearings. I'm pretty sure my old lady wouldn't be into lying to herself like that.

What the self-help people are really referring to is *imagination* and how you can use it to shape your behavior. Without a doubt, imagination is essential for change. You have to conceive of a new behavior or action before you can attempt it. If you never think of looking for a new job or walking a 5K, you'll never do either one.

Stretching your mind allows you to move beyond self-imposed boundaries, but your imagination can also play tricks on you. If you never imagine you're "too fat" to go to the party, you won't end up back in bed with the covers over your head and every stitch of clothing you own on the floor.

Depending what you do with it, imagination can inspire you or pull you under like quicksand. It's formless. It wanders. It can bait you, but, alone, it's too fickle to lead the charge. There are two other crucial elements at play if you want to make change stick: *behavior* (what you do) and *motivation* (the thing that makes you do it).

You begin by perceiving or imagining yourself a certain way—for example: as an athlete or, at the other end of the spectrum, as somebody too tired or stressed to eat well or exercise—and that scenario gets cemented into place by behavior: habitual, repetitive behavior.

But in between imagination and action sits the most important part of the equation: *motivation*—the opaque, widely misunderstood force that drives you to do what you do.

When you're drawn to the refrigerator for the third time after dinner, you are *motivated* to seek out the relief that comes from a late-night food fix, but that kind of scenario is usually identified as "failure," "weakness," or "lack of willpower." Don't be misled. That drive is motivation in its truest form.

At its root, motivation is more like *thirst*. It's an urgent impulse that won't be denied, and like imagination, it cuts both ways. You might thirst for that late-night snack, or if you're a runner by nature, you might thirst for the wind on your face as you sprint downhill on smooth, freshly poured blacktop. It's an ache, not a casual whim. You're "motivated" to quench your thirst, and actions follow.

How we understand and utilize that longing is everything. We don't (and won't) all thirst to go for a brisk jog, but our bodies do thirst to be accessed, transported, and nurtured. Muscles ache to be stretched and utilized, and our cells yearn for nutrients. For authentic wellness—the kind that comes easily and sticks around—we need to tap into that thirst, and use it to our advantage.

We know how to take action physically. We are perfectly capable of lifting a weight or speaking the words, "I'll have the fruit instead of the hash browns." We have the physical ability, but we don't want to. The choices we're "supposed" to make seem too hard. The food doesn't taste as good; exercise seems boring and painful; and there are dozens of "temptations" coming at us every day, too many to conquer all at once.

If you can discover a genuine impulse, something that drives you toward better health in *any* arena that also happens to feel good—if you can pick one and leverage it—you'll have an easy choice in front of you. It's a powerful starting place. Once you know what it feels like to make an effortless, healthy choice like that, one that aligns with your perception of yourself and stems from something you actually enjoy, you'll begin to look for similar opportunities in other areas. There should be easiness within every choice. Even if trying something new presents you with a solid challenge, the effort should feel like a natural outgrowth of who you are and who you're in the process of becoming. As you read on, you'll generate ideas about what some of those options might be.

Runners get off on running. Yogis find their centers in down dog. People who eat well and take care of their bodies feel better because of it. They don't tend to despise the healthy choices they make. It makes no sense to strong-arm ourselves into doing things we hate in order to achieve results we want to love.

All three elements—imagination, thirst, and behavior—need to work together. Imagination is the spark; thirst is the drive; and behavior accumulates to establish the facts of your life and body. All three are there to serve you. You can tug yourself along with one or the other of these elements, but without all three, you won't feel quite right. The changes you make won't be easy, and any progress made will be unlikely to last.

If you can dream it up, enjoy it, follow through and *do it* repeatedly, you will change—and that change will allow you to dream up something else, something new to propel you forward all over again. It's a practice of pursuing small changes that can easily enhance your sense of well-being and lead to newer, bigger, better things.

The first client I ever had was, by far, my most challenging, and I didn't have anywhere near enough experience to help her. She tried to get in shape with behavior alone. Work out, and you'll lose weight, right? A lot of us try to approach our bodies this way. Her method seemed reasonable to me at the time. I figured she'd see results if she exercised enough and ate a little better, no matter her frame of mind. But she taught me the first of many lessons my clients would offer over the years. She strove to change her behavior, but with every step, imagination and thirst held her back, undermining her progress.

Diane was an account executive at a large company, soft-spoken and generous. She was in her forties and about seventy-five pounds overweight. Intensely private, she kept her head low, shrouding her face in long, salt-and-pepper hair and her body in oversized, floor-length skirts she had owned for decades. She resented her body and focused all of her efforts on defeating it.

She signed up for personal training twice a week and performed the exercises I prescribed; but behind every earnest attempt was an unshakable certainty that she was destined to be lonely and obese. She could not imagine that the substance of her life might be malleable. Loneliness, obesity, and her identity were inextricably tied together. She was bulletproof, incapable of imagining the possibility of anything else. She fantasized about a different body, but, like a little girl imagining how to fit into the glass slipper, dreams of finding joy in her body remained in the realm of impossible fantasy.

I was a twenty-four-year-old temp, working the front desk at her company. I received my personal training certification just days before our sessions began, and I'm sure my lack of experience appealed to her. I was overly cautious, unlikely to push her out of her comfort zone, and she appreciated that I was openly riddled with body image issues of my own.

Diane had always struggled with her weight. She moved out of her parents' house at sixteen. She never went to college but worked her way up to a well-respected, high-paying position. She lived alone an hour outside of L.A. and trudged back and forth each day through impenetrable traffic. The details of her early life were murky, but basically, from her teens to the present, she felt abandoned by her family first and men second. Food became a velvet coffin, a cozy, luxurious dead end, too immediately gratifying to leave behind. Food tranquilized her and was always accessible, but the bigger she got, the more isolated and uncomfortable she became. The more judgmental she was of that downward spiral, the more weight she gained.

Most of her days were a wash of work and takeout. She was fiercely loyal to her friends, but she wasn't able to direct any of that compassion toward herself. Thoughts of romance were scarce and, when they did rise up, brought only resignation to a life without companionship. She presumed that most of her struggles came as a direct result of the weight, so she raged against it with liquid diets, over-the-counter pills, and lethargic hours spent at the gym. But in the evening, she found herself at home—another night; another glance at the belly rolls she deemed so disgusting; and another expedition to the white light of the freezer.

Though internally at war, she handled external obstacles with remarkable grace. During our time together, she broke her foot; sprained her knee; underwent multiple surgeries; and three people she loved passed away in quick succession. Through it all, she continued to excel at work, and eventually went to college to pursue an undergraduate degree in English literature for no reason other than because she had always dreamed of doing so.

No one could ever say that her life had been easy, but she possessed powerful wisdom and tenacity. She was smart and ambitious but lacked the most basic belief in her own capacity for wellness. Her life was as she saw it, heavy with ancient baggage and destined for unwanted solitude. The beauty her friends and I saw in her did not jive at all with the way she saw herself. Years passed, slipping through her hands. Her situation was difficult to watch—a person with so much vitality and so much to give defining herself by something as irrelevant as a few pounds of adipose tissue. I tapped at her cellblock of imagination, poking and prodding, cheering and challenging to no avail.

Her only real thirst was for the comfort of chips and cookies, and all of her energy was focused on stopping, quitting, or reducing that thirst. When she was unable to maintain that self-imposed deprivation, she identified as a failure, ate more, exercised more, and maintained her weight just as it was.

We stretched her body a little at a time; strengthened her back; and eased her chronic sciatica. She requested short meditations at the end of each session and, occasionally, was able to let her breath go and her mind rest. I wanted her to feel radiant, but of course, that wasn't up to me. If she couldn't imagine that happiness (or sexiness, for that matter) existed as a possibility for her someday-somehow, no amount of encouragement from me could change that. No matter what I said or did, there was no transformation of her internal narrative.

She couldn't perceive pleasure through the body she so hated. Without any appreciation for the strides she was making or any vision for adventures she might like to explore, the only thing driving her was contempt.

She showed me, first hand, how the assumptions we make about ourselves mold us and forced me to look inward at my own stubborn beliefs—that depression was a way of life for me; that I'd always be chubby and should get comfortable with having a messed up relationship with food because that's just the way it was. I was guilty of equally obstinate thinking and realized that my own friends and family likely saw me as I saw her—full of possibility but hopelessly stuck in a pernicious self-image.

By meeting my encouragement with resistance at every turn, she became a living example of what an impenetrable wall we're capable of building in our own minds and how that wall can directly block forward motion. I wasn't experienced enough to see that the very nature of her fight—her fixed identity in combination with the longing to destroy it— was self-defeating. There was no available path to victory. She was done before she started.

Being overweight is not a purgatory sentence. Millions of people are overweight, strong, and beautiful, but the idea that those attributes could exist simultaneously was beyond Diane's imagination. She couldn't see beauty in the utility of her body as it carried her through her days, and without that basic appreciation, she couldn't find a functional starting place.

In spite of herself, after years of gentle training, her body stood a little taller, her chest a little more open, and the lines in her forehead a little less defined. The regular practice of moving and breathing did have an effect, but she would have seen much greater results if she had allowed herself to recognize the power of incremental progress as it came.

Diane showed me the result of digging in your heels and how much potential can be lost. She never went looking for pleasurable, nurturing activities or food and remained tirelessly fixated on what she *didn't*

want. She had no enthusiasm for where she was headed or acknowledg-
ment of how far she had come. So she went through the motions—
bend-straighten-bend-straighten—and tried and failed to restrict each
morsel she put in her mouth. A bite of brownie was both transcendent
and depraved. The condemnation was constant. Her intentions were
good, but in the end, heartless calisthenics alone couldn't transform
her.

An open mind would have gone a long way. She didn't need to
pretend to be thin. She just needed to feel the length in her back, the
strength in her arms, and to let those new sensations translate to something exquisite, something that indicated her life and body were in the
process of being renewed.

Bodies and minds move in tandem like right and left feet in motion.
One steps forward to bear the weight while the other swings in mid-air,
readying itself to land a few inches ahead of the other. They coax each
other along. If one foot overreaches, total system collapse. And when
we find ourselves in a tangled heap, flat on the ground, it's so easy to
crawl on hands and knees back into an old, familiar place where we're
safe from the hazards of another misstep.

As we come into adulthood, we assemble structures, boxes around
ourselves that define the basics of who we are and limit our understanding of what's possible. They are shelters that, over time, can begin to
function like vaults. Often, we build them at such a young age that we
don't even know they're there. Some are helpful. Maybe you've always
been "the smart one" or "the laid-back one." To some degree, they're
necessary and healthy. They're the backbone of our identities, but when
you find yourself stuck in a box you dislike, unable to get out, the lack of
fresh air can be debilitating. If you wrote yourself off long ago as "the
chubby but funny girl," after five or fifteen years, you might grow tired
of that distinction.

We adopt these "truths" about ourselves and never go back to revisit
them, to consider whether they might be questionable. They hover over

our lives and bore their way into our constitutions: "I suck at sports," "I'm a terrible cook," or the ever popular "I'm too fat for that."

So you find yourself tucked in the box, hugging your knees and staring at the sliver of daylight coming through the intersection where the lid meets the wall. You don't want to be there anymore. Limitation hangs in the air, and it's difficult to breathe. You want fresh air like sustenance, but every time you've tried to escape in the past, it's been a spectacular debacle leaving you beaten and limping back to home base, quietly closing the lid, and snuggling up inside. If that's the case, you probably made one of two missteps.

The first is insurrection: rising up and blasting your way out, cocksure that you're ready to trounce the competition in the Iron Man. You despise the box so much that you attempt to smash it. The whole structure flips on its side, and you find yourself splayed out, blinded by the glare. Your body and mind are stiff from incarceration, and after the initial adrenaline rush subsides, you roll over and quietly draw the lid back to its resting place, out of breath and resigned.

The second misstep is to try to starve or deprive your way out. You don't like it in there but can't seem to escape. You figure the opening isn't big enough for your "fat ass" to squeeze through anyway, so the only option is to make all necessary changes while still sealed inside. You're determined. You do your daily squats in the "fat girl box" but keep banging your head on the lid. The plan is to restrict and control your way out: no sweets, no cheese, no alcohol, and sixty minutes on the elliptical three times a week, plus spin on Tuesdays. This approach is punitive. "I'm stuck. To get out, I'll deny myself all the fun, and if I catch myself having any, I'll make sure to feel bad about it later." It's no way to live, and it backfires with binges of chocolate and chimichangas. "Why," you wonder yet again, "doesn't anything ever work?"

To restrict is defined by Dictionary.com as: "to confine or keep within limits, as of space, action, choice, intensity, or quantity." Confinement suffocates. It leaves you depleted or recalcitrant and sets you up to betray your own self-inflicted boundaries. In combat with yourself, you lash out, diving into a flurry of potato chips and swearing that next time, in the morning, you'll do a better job of denying yourself.

If revitalization of body or mind is your purpose, you can't get there by stifling your natural inclinations or choking down food you hate. Prescribed limitation and forced enthusiasm set you up for failure. They put you en route to a life you wouldn't like, even if you actually managed to get there.

You don't need greater willpower; you need enticement, seduction, something alluring pulling you forward, *toward* a body that thrives. There's a big difference between stepping away from a second bowl of ice cream because you're supposed to and stepping away because you feel better without it. People who succeed in making significant changes have something immediately accessible drawing them toward what they want. It's thirst, not renunciation.

A wise doctor told me once that love and fear are the only two things that change us. Frightening developments like cancer scare people into changing. They fight for survival and do everything in their power to live better and longer. Fear of illness or death can be a remarkable motivator, perhaps the most powerful one there is, but who among us would elect to face that sort of challenge?

There is another way. Passion. Falling in love with feeling better. If you think of times you've been swept away by a wave of enthusiasm—planning a big event; preparing for a career that you love; gaining the attention of a lover; or as a kid, practicing a skill you cared about—when an impulse to act is genuine, it feels effortless, challenging but wholly satisfying.

Reshaping your body and the way you think about fitness can be all of those things if your approach is liberation rather than restriction. We can all wait around for fear to come along and motivate us, but why? Why waste those years when your own fascination with whatever you love has the capacity to pull you up and out?

Find something you enjoy that also makes you healthier and clearer, and do that thing *as often as you can*. That's the first step. It doesn't have to be marathon training. In fact, often the smaller the step, the better. New activities or habits can be challenging, but they should not cause pain or frustration.

Physical activity, no matter how modest, impacts the brain. It sends waves of juicy signals through the neurological system to awaken the mind. Shift your objective to moving and feeding your body *in ways that feel rewarding*. Garden, build a playground, ride a horse, try Tai Chi, or take a walk after dinner every night. Rouse your body to loosen your mind, and your mind will follow.

Begin to recognize what lights you up and what shuts you down. Learn on a visceral level that an overfed, bloated belly before bed feels onerous and a warm, summer sunset with a glass of wine is sublime. You already know the difference. You know what feels heartening or hopeless while you're still in the middle of it. Trust yourself. If you hate it, stop doing it, and try something else instead. Keep looking for the thing that's *your* thing.

Diane neutered her imagination and spent all of her resources trying to dominate her body. In the process, she diminished her spirit. But I've worked with other clients—starting from equally difficult circum-stances—who flourish. They begin with small physical changes that make them feel better and let those changes take root before moving on to bigger, more stimulating ones. They allow their imaginations to wan-der and thirst to grow—for more air, more strength, more clarity of mind. Freedom.

With this new framework comes a simple question: Does what you're doing right now liberate you? Do the activities, foods, and relationships in your life lighten your load or weigh you down? Ask the question in every pocket of your life, and follow it with action—any action, big or small—to support the life and body you want. Do it detective style without judgment, and let your bad habits be what they are while you supplement them with healthier ones.

And if you're worried that removing your usual restrictions will make you act out, eating everything in sight, remember that spinning out of control, bingeing or atrophying on the sofa—is not freeing. Neither is obsessively dieting or overtraining. If you're asking the right question and summoning an honest answer, you'll have no trouble distinguishing restriction from expansion.

If you want something different but don't know how to get there, consider the assumptions you make about yourself and entertain the notion that you might be wrong about them. Something else might be possible.

Who is your old lady, and what has she done all her life that made her who she is? What are some things you assumed "weren't you" that might be second nature to her?

Go after what you love. Lust after the time you spend walking your dog if that's where it starts; lust after watermelon or heirloom tomatoes. Do something concrete. Try a new recipe once a week. Pick one food and one activity to try for one month, and leave it at that. Stop disciplining yourself into submission, and let the rest of your habits play out undisturbed.

Decorate the life you have now—not your ideal life—the one that exists right now, decorate it with food and actions that clear your mind and make your days better.

There will be obstacles, and they will all be very real. We'll address them in detail in the next chapter, but to begin, all there is to do is find a few things that make you stronger—and do them more. Your body, desires, fears, impulses and ambition are all on your side. Leverage them rather than trying to defeat them.

A few years ago, I could not have imagined how remarkable I would feel, stepping out of my front door and taking a walk in the summer heat in a featherweight body. That body and all of the choices required to bring it into being were too far off. To get there, I had to stand up and walk out my door hundreds of other times simply because doing so cleared my head and let me think about things that never would have occurred to me while staring down the barrel of a bag of chips—like starting a business, making a phone call to somebody who could use a familiar voice on the other end, or doing a happy, headphone dance all by myself in the bathroom at the coffee shop for no reason at all.

Once I found my way to the summertime body I craved, I had to stay focused on the tangible behavior that landed me there. Every time I picked up my weapons again and headed back into combat with food or exercise, I began to slip. I became reactionary and obsessed, and the weight crept back on. The fight was feeding the problem, not solving it.

All I really wanted was to feel at ease, body and mind, and that release became the object of my thirst. I ached for peace of mind and a body that felt light, strong, adequately energized, and relatively pain-free. I didn't need six-pack abs or a specific number on the scale anymore. I just wanted to feel well.

Finally, the small decisions that made up my days began to align with that purpose, and when I realized, under streetlights that summer night, that I had accomplished what I set out to do, it felt nothing short of miraculous. But it wasn't miraculous. That triumph was the result of many years of moving, stretching, writing, and breathing my way forward.

I thirsted for better health and something resembling sanity. I got both of those things, but to do that, I had to place value on something other than weight loss and assign blame to something other than my body. I sought out things that turned me on and abandoned—without apology—those that shut me down.

I had plenty more to figure out: how to survive the winter without medicating shortened daylight hours with sugar and how to process heartache or rejection without sabotaging myself. But I finally understood, even at my darkest, that overeating never helped. It just made me numb and heavyhearted. I did it because I didn't know what else to do. I didn't know how else to soothe anxiety or seek pleasure.

If weight loss is your objective, thirsting for healthful things you crave will get you further than any diet ever will. Of course, your diet and activity levels will have to change, but those changes should be a natural outgrowth of a much larger pursuit.

Take better care. Cultivate your thirst. Stretch. Expand. Recoil when necessary. And reach again for things that give you life. It's the only guiding principle you need.

TOOLBOX

What assumptions have you made about yourself that might be worth playing with?
Consider for a second that you might be able to learn to cook a little better or that sweating might not be the end of the world if you can chat with a friend while you do it. Maybe you don't have to be witty all the time. Maybe you could wear glasses or chop off your hair. Throw your identity up in the air, and let it scatter. Fifty-two card pickup. See which cards are worth gathering up again and which aren't.

Choose one activity you always wanted to do but never did, and give it a try.
Coax your imagination. Think of activities that have piqued your interest but were never pursued because they seemed far-fetched or you simply didn't make them a priority. Make a list of fantasies and adventures big and small, and look through them to see if there are scaled down versions you could explore. If you love the idea of Diana Nyad swimming from Cuba to Florida, see if there is a river or lake in your town that you could safely conquer. If you want to learn to cook, invite a friend over once a week to help you try out a new recipe.

Figure out what you already love that is both healthy and gratifying.
Find your thirst. Make a list of all of the healthy food and activities that you also happen to love. You can turn to anything on this list when life gets chaotic and you lose touch with the pursuit of wellness—from blueberries to fresh whole grain bread, from gardening to dancing, from evening walks to roller-skating. If you're writing this list in your journal, leave an extra page or two blank at the end knowing that it will

continue to expand over time as you realize how many things you thirst for that also happen to be healthy.

Choose one of those healthy habits to reintroduce on a daily or weekly basis.

From your list, choose one thing that you love but had forgotten about, and bring it back into your life on a regular basis. Just pick one for now, and make it a really easy one, something fun or yummy that won't take up too much time or cost too much money. Decide on a schedule, and do it regularly. You can write down the date every time it happens at first or put it on a calendar if you need extra reinforcement.

Does what you are doing right now lighten your load or weigh you down?

Begin asking yourself this question throughout your day to heighten your awareness of what is and is not helpful for your body and your life. If you're eating too much on a regular basis, spend some time noticing how that makes you feel physically in the moment and afterward. Notice both the good and the bad, but don't worry about changing any of it yet. Just take a look at it. That awareness will become a crucial part of the process of getting better.

3

DAY AND NIGHT

I met a new client recently who came through the door of my gym full of idealistic goals and numbers, tactics and techniques for weight loss. She perched on the edge of my weight bench, with her back self-consciously turned to the mirror, and told me a familiar story of unmet ambition.

She had a laundry list of diets she had tried and workouts she planned to try next. She hoped to get a quick answer, a static plan to take with her. I inquired about her family history, her relationship with food and exercise as a teenager, her work life, and the nagging habits that frustrated her most. She answered and shifted on the bench before turning her gaze up and closing her eyes to a rush of tears.

This happens all the time on my little bench. It's not a comfortable place to sit. There's nothing to lean against, nothing to fiddle with or fall back on, no pillows to conceal laps, bellies, and thighs. It's just a bench, but it has a tendency to lay things bare.

Her tactics weren't working. They never really had. As she reviewed her situation out loud for my benefit, she realized that all the effort she put in over the course of many years had won her nothing at all. She wasted an undeniable amount of time, and here she was, sitting on a bench, facing the same body she had begun battling years earlier—only now, twenty-five pounds heavier.

She came through my door that day immersed in something I call *cheerleader mindset*. Optimistic and open-hearted, earnest and energetic, she got up every morning ready to conquer her cravings and lose the weight. In spite of feeling perpetually in a state of failure, she continued to believe "I can do this; I can do it *this* time." She set her mind to it. Chin up. Focused. Poised for success. But every "failure" brought another slow bleed of her confidence. She gave her all: every night, every New Year's Eve, a new plan, a new effort—but the constant strategizing was all for nothing. And here she was again, this time acknowledging the tsunami of lost potential, the energy she had wasted imprisoning the body she could have been working to free.

It's easy, from a cool distance, to say that wellness and weight loss are best achieved by getting back in touch with your body and going after things that turn you on, but what about the bad habits that seem unbreakable? What about the relentless late nights that seem to undo every productive, healthy day?

In theory, you can say you'll make a better choice next time, but how does that actually happen? How do better decisions get made time and again until they add up to a fitter body and a mind that has more valuable things to think about than how many calories are in a pat of butter?

Trying to overcome ingrained impulses by telling yourself how weak and worthless you are clearly doesn't work. Diligent, sensible planning doesn't work either. The impulses are too demanding, too sweetly distracting. Bad habits persist, and tough times come. We can all count on death and taxes, right? But if we allow those tough times to chip away at our health, it makes everything so much harder to handle.

The only sustainable option is to figure out how to use the challenges we face to *deepen* our wellness as we go. Use them like you own them—because you do.

Instead of trying to fight off bad habits, what if we let them come and spend some time noticing how they actually impact us? Once we can see and feel them for what they are, it's so much easier to reach for something different. Nobody wants to feel bad. If framed correctly, our destructive habits can be engines for change. They can be employed to secure their own demise.

There are two distinct and reliable mindsets vying for control of your behavior day and night. The *Cheerleader* is the first. She is with you upon waking (or after your first cup of caffeine). She fights to hold off destructive impulses all day, putting her best face forward. By dusk, on the drive home from work, her energy is spent, and she closes her eyes to rest until dawn.

You sink into the driver's seat and coast. Your shoulders begin to release. The muscles around your eyes soften as daylight dims and the easy shield of night arises. With that, the second mindset arrives, a shadowy figure I have affectionately come to refer to as *Lothario*.

Throughout history, Lothario has been defined as a lascivious character, a gentleman caller who plays upon the weaknesses of the women he seduces. When the Cheerleader begins to drift off, Lothario appears in the backseat. He strokes your neck with both hands as you drive. He traces the arc of your shoulders, down the crease of your elbows, before placing his hands firmly over your own and interlacing his fingers with yours around the steering wheel. He guides you ever so smoothly to turn to the right, directly into the parking lot of the Winn Dixie.

With no fight left in you, you surrender. The steps to the ice cream section, the phone call to the pizza guy, and the spoon buried in the pint are all foregone conclusions before you ever set foot in your home. When the Cheerleader runs out of steam (which she always does), Lothario is waiting, and his arrival is a welcome relief. He eases your mind for the night, filling you with distraction and momentary satisfaction before tucking you into bed. He pulls the covers to your chin and leaves you drugged by the sleepy effects of salt, sugar, fat, and a nice cabernet.

When you wake up in the morning, the Cheerleader rubs her eyes. She's confused by the bloated belly that arrived overnight but shakes it off and sets out again to conquer the day—one step forward, one step back.

We pit Lothario and the Cheerleader against one another in battle, but why? Lothario's purpose is to soothe. His greatest aspiration is to give you a break from the hyper-vigilance of your day, which is not bad in and of itself. The Cheerleader's purpose is to uplift, to make you healthier and mitigate the damage done by Lothario's late-night seductions. Both mean well. Neither means harm, but we invariably glorify one and attempt to subjugate the other.

If the Cheerleader could relax a little and stop shooting for perfection; if she could pay attention to what makes your body feel more alive rather than what will beat it into shape as fast as possible, Lothario wouldn't have to bust out a box of cookies after dinner to help you recover from the beat-down. And if Lothario didn't have to indulge every unhealthy whim to make you feel satisfied and relaxed, the Cheerleader wouldn't have to overcompensate to recover.

There are a million, perfectly valid reasons why we indulge in behavior that does us no good. Work is hard; dating is annoying; the kids are unruly. We face anxiety, restlessness, and boredom. Lovers leave, and people die. It makes sense that we want to tranquilize some of it. We need a break. We yearn to lay down the load, and Lothario is happy to oblige. The problem is that we aren't turning to the right release valves.

Working against each other, the Cheerleader and Lothario will always clash. The Cheerleader pushes for all-or-nothing, and Lothario is too robust to deny. But when united for the same cause, when pleasure and wellness *merge*, the results can be astonishing. There is suddenly no need for blunt force effort to keep going, and unhealthy cravings can naturally subside. We need them to work together so indulgence and health can spring from the same source.

I don't come by this information easily, by the way. I fully understand how difficult it is to break out of a rut. I know how disturbing it is to feel like your body is a weird, ill-fitting suit that you can't take off. I get it. I've been there. Fortunately, the methods that lifted me up and out are accessible to anyone who wants them, and they begin in a place you're probably all too familiar with—right smack in the middle of the frustration.

When I first realized the consuming force Lothario wielded in my own life, I decided to let him have his way. I was too tired to fight him off. My Cheerleader was beat. She was lying down on the job. The decision to curl up willingly in his arms was a last resort, but I knew I didn't have the strength to defeat him. I knew I was in a losing battle, and if I was going to give in anyway, I figured I might as well luxuriate in the comfort.

At first, giving over to him felt like falling off the edge of a cliff. It was terrifying to imagine what might happen to my body if I let my worst impulses run rampant, but that willingness to relax into the mess, without trying to fix it turned out to be the best and only thing I could have done to begin getting better.

I was living in New York City, marinating in depression, twenty-two, and newly graduated from college. I was supposed to be on my honeymoon in a log cabin in Kauai, but three weeks before our wedding, my fiancé of two years dumped me via voice mail. Invitations had been sent, plane tickets had been bought, and portraits had been taken of me standing in ivory lace at my parents' hearth. The heartbreak was driven home by sudden, public humiliation and topped off with a blow, bone-deep, to my confidence.

I was blindsided and couldn't comprehend what was going on inside the mind of this man I thought I had known so intimately. If I couldn't be sure of the love he had showered on me, I couldn't be sure of anything. He had made me feel like I was sitting in a rocking chair on God's front stoop, bathed in sunlight under the steady gaze of my beloved's clear blue eyes. But he was gone. With him went my enthusiasm and, even worse, the ability to rely on my own judgment.

I sought help from a therapist who made sure I was stable, but the depression was unyielding. It had been nipping at my heels since my late teens, and fighting it seemed like a waste of time. I ate in secret, stopping in at bodegas, pizza parlors, and burrito stands. I was anonymous in such a huge city and gratefully disappeared into the masses, hiding on street corners, eating in a vain attempt to buoy my spirits as waves of grief came and went. I sublet a room in an apartment full of functional people and went to bed.

The city was dirty and crowded to match my mood. There were old buildings and certifiable neighbors screaming at phantoms at all hours of the night. There were rats in the subway, buskers on the street, and cheap socks in Chinatown.

Days and nights passed. I temped and cocktail waitressed. I stared at the bathroom mirror; blinked at the street outside; dug stacks of Chips Ahoy! and Twix bars out of the far reaches of my closet; crawled back into bed; and waited for something to happen. I hated my body, hated food, and lost all faith in truth and honesty.

It's difficult to remember depression accurately. Sadness is part of it, of course, but beyond that, there is a heaviness, a stiffness and ache that encroaches on the body. Inertia takes over, and your muscles and bones feel like they are beginning to atrophy and die. Days and weeks stretch out ahead, a marathon of empty initiative. But there is beauty there too, satisfaction. The despair becomes an uncomplicated resting place to return to. And, for me, food was there to smooth over the whole mess, sticky and sweet.

In my most insane moments I had a fantasy that I could chop off the edges of my thighs with a kitchen knife. Attractive, I know, but so easy to fit into jeans then, right?! But, alas, that wasn't a reasonable option, so I turned to whatever distractions might help me through the night: food, sleep, alcohol, movies—whatever. I let Lothario bring every creature comfort he could and curled up appreciatively in his embrace.

I didn't recognize until much later that the instinct that alerted me to the insanity of carving off my thighs with the kitchen knife was, in an odd way, the same life-giving one that would guide me to my feather-weight body almost a decade later. Humans have an instinct to survive—and to survive we need to maintain our health as best we can, which does not, in case you were wondering, include shaving off the edges of your thighs with a kitchen knife.

We know what feels right or wrong with regards to survival. We know not to cut through a dark alley alone. We feel uneasy when reaching too high on an unstable ladder, and stepping back is a relief, not an obligation. This simple survival instinct drives us to stay safe and agile, but, ironically, it's the same reason we eat to medicate stress. Our brains recognize that eating provides us with extra energy reserves for stressful situations. Food is reinforcement—until we overeat and become too heavy to outrun the theoretical lions on the ancestral plain.

You can feel the switch happening—from nourishing, helpful eating to impulsive, destructive eating—but it's a quiet hum, not a blaring alarm. Faint pings of discomfort alert you when enough is enough, when one more slice of pizza will make you feel worse, not better. The shift is hard to sense at first, but that basic knowing is there at your disposal. The same can be said for exercise. The right amount feels great, but too much or too little feels wrong. The instinct to stay light and strong is present, but minding it is so much easier said than done.

For the time being, perched in limbo in New York, I allowed food to be a comfort. I ate because I was sad. Sweetness, fat, and salt made me feel "better," and in those moments, I needed relief more than anything else. From there, I went looking for my best instincts, the ones I had lost track of, faint pings telling me what might make my body feel a little better.

Early on in that search, I came across a lecture by a psychologist and teacher named Ram Dass (also known as Richard Alpert of Harvard University). He offered an intriguing place to begin.

He told a story about a woman he barely knew who called him in the middle of the night threatening suicide. She was barely coherent, so he asked her (I'm paraphrasing here), "Who was it that picked up the phone and dialed eleven numbers to get me on the other line? I would like to speak with *that* person, the functional part of you that physically picked up the phone and dialed."[1]

After talking her down, he asked her to imagine a painting of a large, dark cloud filling the majority of a picture frame with a small sliver of clear, blue sky peeking out from the corner—the only way to discern that it was a cloud in the first place. That little bit of blue sky was the functional part of the woman that picked up the phone.

He called it "the witness," the part of her that could objectively observe her own experience, a neutral perspective, a calm awareness on the outside of the drama that could allow a crack of daylight into an otherwise pitch-dark room.

I began to cultivate that idea, staying at least a little aware of the fact that I was eating a giant veggie burger, fries, and half a dozen doughnuts while I was still in the throes of doing it. No judgment, no fight. Just, "Hey, look at that. There I go again." I wasn't trying to control the behavior. I was just observing it and watching how it impacted me. Whether I kept eating or not didn't matter, as long as I stayed aware of the taste, the grease, the numb satisfaction, and even deeper sadness that followed.

I went in search of my little bit of blue sky anywhere and everywhere I could, and after a time, I began searching for something even greater than neutrality. I started searching for tiny shards of joy that might be scattered throughout the days and nights, noting them and letting them in.

As summer turned to fall, I made a few choices with forward momentum. I got out of bed and went to the park to look at the space between the leaves where the sun came through. Walking to or from work, feeling like my nutrition-deprived body might give out on the relentless stretches of concrete, I passed cathedrals with open doors and went inside to the cool darkness to sit in a place where silence was constant. I spent time cuddled up with every dog or cat who would have me; and danced at clubs until four in the morning, accompanied by flamboyant compatriots who didn't seem to mind one way or the other how fat or thin I was. I found a rhythm in the city, doing whatever I could to discover how to feel again, how to see and hear and be touched again.

It was an honest state of being. I didn't spend my mornings pretending that I would be able to control my eating at night. I knew what was coming and let it be. At least, in Lothario's arms, I could relax. Even if my belly ballooned, I could lay back and look up in search of the sky between the clouds.

Small things began to soothe my urge to eat for comfort. I was inadvertently building behavior that would eventually free me from a heavy heart, dependence on food, and festering hatred for my body. Most of the time, I still abused food, but bubbling up from under that abuse was an urgent aspiration to experience my body in a new way and a distant belief that I had a shot—that someday it might be possible to get through a whole day without a litany of my faults and failures running through my brain on auto-repeat. Big dreams, they were. I was making way for open space and wanted more.

I began adding as many healthy habits as I could manage into the chaos, peppering it with lightness. Instead of trying to put out destructive fires, I started feeding healthy ones.

I have no idea what caused me to start resenting my body and relying on food for solace in the first place. Those toxic habits were with me long before the broken engagement and depression. The heartache just made them worse. There were probably many causes over the years. All I knew was that when times were tough, eating made me feel better, and when life was pretty good, I kept right on eating anyway. Food was reliable, and I used it daily to dull boredom, loneliness, aimlessness, and panic.

I never did figure out what caused it, but eventually I decided that *it didn't matter*. Fixating on the past and trying to put together a puzzle with missing pieces was not working, so I gave up. Striving to know the unknowable was not getting me anywhere. The past was what it was. There was nothing I could do to change it. It was too vast, exhausting, and far away. All that mattered was finding a way to get better, starting now.

I realized with blinds drawn against broad daylight that I had a lot of years to go, and I had a choice to make. I could get worse, or I could get better. I could drift further away from life or reach for it in whatever small way I could muster.

There's not a soul in the world, not a compliment from a lover, and not a lie you tell yourself that can mask the truth of how your body feels under your hands in the dead of night. That silent space is yours alone. But it *is* possible for that silence to be permeated by awareness instead of failure. Discomfort can inform you rather than defeat you, if you let it.

Based on my own experience and that of my clients, I have to suggest you try something a bit unorthodox, something you wouldn't expect any self-respecting personal trainer or self-helpy-type author to ever recommend: *Do the thing that makes you feel like crap, and then do it again.* Wrap your life around it for a while before you attempt to make any change at all. Get intimate with exactly how you feel after eating too much or not moving enough. Do it for however long it takes until you know in your bone marrow that you don't want to feel like that anymore. That knowledge—fully understood in your gut and stiff, aching muscles—is fuel that will propel you to a different way of life and a body that moves and breathes with ease.

I have to qualify this instruction with a plea for your safety: If your impulses are leading you to do anything that puts you or anybody else in harm's way, obviously, don't do it. Talk to somebody. Seek help. There are counselors and agencies available for free to help you handle depression and destructive impulses.[2]

But if you're just plain unhealthy, frustrated, and trying to get better, think of these visits to the dark side as useful reminders, not obstacles to overcome. Discover and register them instead of shutting them out. Without them you would be lost in a netherworld of feeling vaguely lousy with no clear way out. They give you something very specific to work with. That feeling of yuck alerts you when nasty habits have crept in to play therapist again.

As you work with this, you'll begin to catch them earlier. You'll recognize when bad habits are about to sneak up on you, and, with the help of later chapters in this book, you'll have fallback systems in place to help you get past them before too much damage is done. When you catch them coming, you'll know exactly what to do. You'll figure out how to counteract early-warning behavior rather than having to rely on crisis management. The systems you use to ward off bad habits and to support the active growth of new, good ones will be one and the same. There will be one unified process moving you forward, accessible at any time no matter how well or badly any given day is going. But to start utilizing that process, you have to be able to recognize what's happening *as it's happening*, and start interrupting it.

It's counterintuitive to think that allowing negative impulses to play themselves out might prove helpful. Everybody's always beating the drum of positive thinking. Positive thinking is lovely but pointless if you've lost track of what feels right: how it feels to treat your body well and—even more importantly—how it feels to treat it badly.

Allow yourself to wallow a little. Stop struggling against the mess and take a big, ol' belly flop straight into it. Consider what life would be like if none of it ever changed. How would it feel to live in the body you have now for the rest of your life? How would that body feel to you as you age? Spending time in that space and getting real about what it physically feels like to let unhealthy habits wash over you will help you make more clear-headed decisions about what to do next.

If you can make peace with your body and habits as they are, do it. Spare yourself the struggle. Put energy into respecting your body and caring for it, rather than trying to change it.

But if you decide you want something different, do the destructive things you do as usual, but *as you do*, take note of how it feels to come to, with crumbs on your belly, sickness in your heart, and a pit in your stomach. Notice how it all feels from an objective, judgment-free point of view, and begin supplementing that discomfort with small, specific behavioral changes to make things better.

Go on a quest to discover what makes you feel weighed down, how often it happens, and how bad it gets. The habits themselves will begin to remind you why you don't want to engage in them anymore. There's no point in berating and belittling yourself. Don't bother. It does nothing but add fuel to the wrong fire. Just let it be.

Overeating isn't your worst enemy. Apathy is; blacking out with a bucket of wings is. Sharpen your awareness of how bad habits affect you until you can't stand it anymore. Because if you don't really care that much—if your stomachache, backache, or inability to enjoy the summer sun on your legs aren't bad enough to matter, there's no good reason to shoot for anything better.

Be willing to note what's happening with enough regularity to learn exactly how much you don't want to continue anymore. Get cozy with the negative sensations, and don't try to make any changes at first. Sink in to how you feel in the moment and the following day. Face the physical fallout of your choices with eyes wide open. Throw flour on the ghost, and invite it to stay for cupcakes.

My clients show me all the time what it looks like to persevere and self-destruct at the same time. They leap too hard, too fast. They fail, beat themselves up, and do it all again—but over time, they begin to see that there is a much better way to take care of themselves, to achieve bodies that feel good to them. They can let weight loss evolve out of the goodness in their lives, rather than looking for goodness in their lives to come from weight loss. They can shift their focus from stripping themselves down to building themselves up.

Everybody can find something to appreciate. Even if it's the unhealthy food itself, at least it's there for you when you turn to it. Go ahead and be appreciative of that illicit relief, but pay attention—without judgment—to the discomfort it creates in other areas of your life. If you give yourself a little space to observe the negative repercussions without beating yourself up along the way, you'll be surprised by how quickly that food begins to feel more repulsive than alluring.

And while you're waiting for that lightbulb to come on, if you can step out of your ordinary surroundings and explore a bit, something new will catch your attention and get you moving forward, distracting you in a wonderful way and driving your thirst.

Too much food and no exercise at all should start to look just as damaging and irrational as the kitchen knife. Steps from that place of clarity are tangible. The habits and structure you build to support your new thirst for feeling better and stronger will be straightforward and always accessible. And the questions at the end of each chapter will help you come up with ideas for what can be done right now, at this very moment, with the body you currently have to start quenching that thirst.

The whole metamorphosis begins with compassion. When you fall prey to a bad habit, feeling guilty or pissed about it will only drive you to repeat the behavior. That's how addiction works, whether you're talking about sugar or heroin. The object of your desire soothes you, before torturing you, before soothing you again.

If you can observe the habit and remember that your body and mind are just using a reliable, tried-and-true method to get by, you'll give yourself space to judge the habit on its merits. Is it helping or hurting you? That's all that matters. How exactly does it feel? Once you can see patterns repeating, you (and your Cheerleader) can take concrete action; one step, one system at a time.

There's a recovery center in Nashville called Magdalene, "a residential program for women who have survived lives of prostitution, trafficking, addiction and life on the streets."[3] The women live and work together. They make a line of natural bath and body products that are sold nationwide called Thistle Farms. Everything is manufactured and marketed at their headquarters, on their turf, by their people. It's an extraordinary program.

The women are provided with a support system: housing, health care, therapy, work, and educational training. Every one of these resources helps them build new lives, but before a new arrival can construct a new perception of herself and a fresh way of engaging with the world, she has to show up for the things that matter most: showers, meals, meetings, and work. She has to be willing to let go of survival tactics that might have sustained her on the streets but are now blocking her way. Only then can she build new ones that support a different experience.

I don't bring these women up to cast aspersions on the rest of us who have an easier life, to imply that we shouldn't be complaining about our bodies or lack of time. We all struggle in our own way, and none of it is easy.

I bring them up because their example shows how to get down to basics. They have seen and experienced the worst of the worst. They know exactly how difficult life can get. To extricate themselves from a life of suffering and abuse, they learn how to stop judging themselves for the past and start doing what needs to be done, no matter how small or insignificant the new habits might seem. They make the necessary structural changes, and those who are able to stick with it discover that little things have an enormous impact. In the end, they find comradery, self-sufficiency, and the holy grail—a resting place in their own hearts.

Give yourself a break. Start where you are, and try something new. It's really the only option you have, and giving yourself a break does not mean surrender. Your daily decisions are not a game of win or lose, all or nothing. The best way to cease the struggle once and for all is to get in touch with your own, sustaining survival instincts, your thirst for something stimulating. Health feels good, and the process of *getting* healthy should feel good too. Every time you catch yourself thinking about belly fat or the new diet everyone is on, step aside. Go looking for a little bit of blue sky anywhere you can find it. Move more, and eat something good. Over time, the goodness will grow, and you will find yourself in a body that feels infinitely better.

Lightness springs from devotion to people and pastimes you love, not from deprivation. In my opinion, living well should always include chocolate and dancing; sunshine and puppies; leather and lace; heartbreak, ridiculousness, and risk.

Night comes. Let it. Dance with Lothario until you're crystal clear what you do and don't want to feel like, and give the Cheerleader a new task. Put her in charge of figuring out what you love that also happens to feed you, body and soul—and do more of those things, many more of them, as often as you can.

TOOLBOX

What makes you feel like crap?

Take a minute to consciously identify which habits or patterns are your worst. Take stock of your day from beginning to end. Are your mornings rushed? Do you eat breakfast? Do you plow through your day on coffee and break room pastries? Do you make questionable choices at lunch? Are you tired in the afternoon? Do you stop for takeout on the way home? How much sugar do you eat? Is there any movement or exercise in your day? Do you have nagging aches and pains? Do you eat or drink too much at night? Getting enough sleep?

You're looking for behavioral patterns that reliably make you feel uncomfortable, lethargic, or stiff. You have to be aware of this stuff before you can do anything about it.

Once you've done that, set the big ones aside and think about your *little* bad habits. If a few of those changed, you'd be surprised what might reverberate on a larger scale. An example: I used to have a miniature peppermint patty after lunch thinking that it was a low-calorie way to get my sweet fix, but I realized at some point that that little hit of pure sugar was making me sleepy and sluggish in the afternoon, leading to unhealthy dinner choices and late-night snacking. Changing that one behavior easily dropped five hundred calories from my days.

Look for small habits that might make a big difference, and don't worry about changing them yet. This step is about recognition and identification. No muss, no fuss.

What makes you feel amazing in your daily life?

Look for glimpses of daylight anywhere you can find them. Make a mental note when one pops up to surprise you: from your cat making you laugh to an unexpected word of encouragement from a friend; from a full moon to an act of kindness you see at your kid's school. As you take active notice of those cracks in the clouds, they will become more obvious and frequent. They'll open up your days. With each little lift, good decisions are easier to make.

If you want to make a journal exercise out of it, write down three things at the end of each day that brought you joy. No matter how difficult dealing with life or food might seem, there are always slivers of blue sky. Make a practice of looking for them and appreciating them for the breath of fresh air that they are.

Continue reinforcing the one healthy habit you added in chapter 2.
Don't forget. Stick with it, and if that one isn't working for you, pick something else. Add another one if you feel like it would be easy to maintain.

4

DIG THE RIDE

Every once in a while, you meet someone who seems at rest in her body. You know it when you see it. There is an unmistakable nonchalance about her, an okay-ness with being as she is. Hanging on to self-consciousness in her presence feels awkward and wrong, like there's just no good reason for it.

These liberated people aren't any different from the rest of us. They're not immune to difficulties or bad habits, but they have mastered one very important skill. They've learned to dig the ride, and it's a beautiful thing to behold.

If we let them, they can be valuable teachers. They come in every shape and size, every color and age. They are almost never six-foot bombshells with beach-tousled hair, dewy lips, and willowy limbs. They're apples and pears like everybody else, but they don't spend much time fretting about how they look. They know how to be open-hearted, even in the face of heavy burdens, but would almost certainly brush you off if you claimed they had any particular insight to share. They know how to celebrate the small things, fully and whole-heartedly, that everybody else takes for granted, and they drive right back into life no matter what obstacles rise up along the way.

They will lure you out of your lair with promises of road trips and ice cream sundaes. They'll coerce you into going to the park for an impromptu amateur photography class, or beg for help running a yard sale to benefit a local dog rescue. In their own lives, they'll make you dizzy as they navigate options you never would have considered, hopping deftly and precariously from one unexpected lily pad to another, never in the same direction, never where you would have expected, but always with levity and peacefulness at the center of their directional equation.

They aren't confident and full of adventure because they're thin. They're lumpy just like the rest of us, but don't seem to care. They see their bodies as useful vehicles, capable of carrying them, and they'll take the ride anywhere because they know all too well that slamming on the brakes is futile.

I've made a habit of looking for these people and following them around like an eager pupil. One such woman is Mignon Francois, a friend of mine who started a small business called the Cupcake Collection with her family in 2008. Mignon has what her mother refers to as a "Kool-Aid" smile. "I show all forty-seven of my teeth when I smile because I've got a lot of smiling to do," she says, "I got a lot of stuff to smile about."[1] Her enthusiasm is infectious and she approaches everything and everyone with love. It oozes out of her.

"We started the business out of necessity," she says. "I needed to find something to do to save my family. We were drowning in debt, drowning in brokenness. We were the working poor, and we set out to start a business that was about comfort, comfort that people could access. When people are down, they come and see me for cupcakes, but it's about so much more than cupcakes for me. It's about healing. It's about renewal."

When she recently discovered that one of her teenage daughters was pregnant, she put on "sackcloth and ashes, the new millennium style" for several painful days of regret and fear before stretching her heart wider and questioning why she was mourning the creation of a new life, a new little family member, one more person to love. When the baby arrived, Mignon's smile grew even wider, as if that were possible.

What began as a bake sale out of her living room has grown into a booming family business with two locations and international press—

and for it all, she is nothing but grateful. She's a walking celebration of life, along for the ride, spreading joy every which way she can in the form of luscious, little cupcakes.

She has given birth to six children and adopted one more "by default." She told me the seventh showed up in need of a family, and happily never left. Mignon's body is sturdy, average-sized, but built to hold the enormity of her heart and to bear the trials and triumphs of poverty and perseverance. Knowing her has changed my understanding of what beauty and success look like, and it has deepened my conviction that sweets can be healing, if used for good. She has no plans to shrink her body or her imprint on the world. She's here to remind those of us who might forget that caring for ourselves means *taking pleasure* in family, friends, and food. Life doesn't get much better than wandering aimlessly into her shop in Germantown, Tennessee, on a Sunday afternoon.

I've been blessed to know a few women like this. Some become dear friends; others I just hold in my mind as lifelines, living reminders of how to stay open and alive. Each has shown me in her own way, through her own life, how to keep moving toward a healthy body no matter what wreckage I'm facing and how to stay nimble in the face of frustration.

They understand that being hyper-vigilant and overly controlling only makes everything stiffer and more likely to break. There is nothing inherently permanent about hard times or the state of our bodies. There's no reason the past has to define the future. If we support them rather than fighting them, our bodies can be at their own, individual versions of best, whatever physical or financial limitations we face.

These women see hardships for what they are. They're not in denial. They might have broken hearts now and then, but they can see their boundaries. No matter where they are, high or low, they understand that beyond any given moment, there is more life to come, a whole lot more living at their fingertips, which might turn out to be good, bad, or interesting. Whatever comes, they stay in motion through it all. Ecstatic or hurting, they are always willing to step back into the driver's seat to see what's around the bend—because there is always something new around the bend.

It's a long ride, and they take no issue that part of it will be tough. When things get scary, instead of clamping down, they arch their backs with arms spread wide and bodies open to whatever comes next. Cellulite and muscle come together as part of one magnificent, whole self doing life. They dodge and weave and try another way. There is curiosity and motion—always forward motion.

Before I began learning from these beautiful souls, I tried to control everything (especially food) to manage stress—but, of course, the best-laid plans never do pan out. My new friends taught me how to roll with the punches. They carved looseness into my life and eventually into my relationship with my body. They taught me to meander my way to a body and mind that work for me.

There are no straight lines from here to there, only squiggly ones—but that's half the fun. I had to study how to dig the ride in the body I had, especially when the going got rough, and I can trace the lines of this liberated body directly back to two specific women, two liberated souls who showed me how it's done through their own living examples.

The first is Sophia. I met her one afternoon while folding my laundry in a friend's living room. She burst through the front door, collapsed on the couch, and began sobbing in a way you never want to witness in a stranger.

She gasped for air while telling us that her lover of ten years had been cheating on her for over a year. She was shuddering from the shock, a mass of long, auburn curls stuck to the side of her face. She could hardly see for swollen eyes or speak for cracked, bleeding lips. She was wrung out.

I had forgotten what it was like to cry like that. As the years passed, my depression had been replaced by vague insecurity and dissatisfaction, but her agony was familiar, a little too familiar. I packed up my things and left them there. They were old friends, and it was not my place to stay.

A few months later, I got an unexpected Christmas present from Sophia. I hadn't seen her since that heartbreaking afternoon, but we had several friends in common and ran in the same circles. I was surprised to receive the box and carefully opened the glittery silver paper to discover that this woman I had met *one* time during one of the most painful moments of her life had bought me a giant, hot pink dildo for Christmas. Actually it was a vibrator, but the word dildo is way more fun to write, so let's go with that.

In her grief one Friday afternoon, she glided into the Hustler store on Sunset Boulevard, wearing a black feather boa, and proceeded to buy dildos for everyone she thought could use some more fun. Clearly this was a woman I needed to know better.

Sophia is a leprechaun dancing in fields of dandelions. She is mischievous and playful. She isn't a small person, physically or otherwise. When she needs to fall apart, she falls apart big, but on the rebound she is unstoppable.

Our friendship grew fast. We were each hurting in our own way and in search of relief, but as I wallowed and tried to shrink, she stretched bigger and wider. I would be moping around on a Saturday afternoon, feeling sorry for myself, and the phone would ring, "Do what you want!" she would say, "Up to you. Sit around by yourself all night, or come see Cindy Lauper with me and drink wine and eat kettle corn. She might be old, but I bet she's still got rainbows in her hair!" This was not a difficult choice.

Sophia would never hold it against me if I turned her down. She would happily call someone else, and that wouldn't stop her from reaching out again the next day or the following weekend to see if I wanted to come along for some other adventure. There was no judgment, just an offer of glee and hilarity if I chose to accept it. Her ability to keep living large, no matter what struggles she might be facing, was astonishing to me.

She was fine with being single in a way I was totally unfamiliar with. My sense of balance in the world and, even more, my day-to-day feelings about my body hinged directly on whether I was in a romantic relationship, the chosen one, physically desired by somebody else. But here was a woman who had no concern that she needed a relationship to make her life complete. She had just been shattered by love, but her solution to the pain was not to hide away. No, the solution was retro Cindy Lauper, Lenny Kravitz, Willie Nelson, Amos Lee, Jack White, and, oh what the hell, while we're at it, Mexico!

We spent six years out on the town until I moved away. Concerts and movies, dancing and hiking, parties with fancy folks at her boss's house in Bel Air, theater and comedy clubs, weekend trips to Vegas and Big Bear. We were living a *Laverne and Shirley* episode.

She lost her job. I temped. She liquidated ten years of shared possessions. I broke my arm on a roller-skating date with a douchebag. This, that, and the other. There was always something happening, some up or down to be had, but every Sunday night, we pulled it together, just the two of us, for dinner and wine at her place—an evening of HBO and okay-ness.

In her home, I ate without shame for the first time in my adult life, and it felt like a miracle. Until then, even with friends and family, I was always assessing how much I should or shouldn't eat, how it might look, what people would think, or how fat I would get. With Sophia, the food that had always caused me such anxiety became a celebration of friendship, a reason to come together.

Before I could learn how to take better care of my body, I had to make friends with it. I had to learn how to enjoy food and be at rest in my skin, in a room with another human being.

Sophia made it easy to be easy.

I told her horrifying things that were swirling around in my head. I wrote a murder ballad about a guy I was dating and performed it for her in her living room. She proclaimed it genius, and we roasted him over the flames. I handed over my heaviest thoughts, and she disintegrated them in her force field. She made every problem seem both completely understandable and utterly ridiculous. She absorbed it all, loved me no matter what, and was always prepared to distract me with a joint or a jig.

Sophia had weight issues of her own. She was fifty or sixty pounds overweight. She wasn't blind to it, but her weight never affected her sense of self-worth or enjoyment of life. She took good care of herself and would have preferred to lose weight, but the extra pounds didn't rule her like they did me. It didn't destroy her relationships or make her feel any less beautiful. Sophia glowed; her body was an enthusiastic expression of who she was, not something to be escaped. Instead of trying to make herself smaller, she adorned herself with bold, colorful jewelry and fabulous, discount shoes.

She was much bigger than me, and as I watched her move through the world, lighthearted and irreverent, I started to feel like a fool for spending so much energy disparaging my body at the cost of my quickly passing twenties. She taught me an obvious fact: life can be magnificent at any size. And she taught me that when all else fails, when the world looks like it's coming to an end, do a little something for somebody else. Buy a dildo for someone in need.

My insecurities didn't disappear in a magical poof of Sophia-smoke, but they were dwarfed by my new friend's love of life and alleviated by my willingness to go with her, along for the ride.

Many years later, in another lifetime and another city, I had been working as a personal trainer for five years. I wasn't a full-blown wreck anymore with regard to my body but was still mired in die-hard habits of worrying about and bargaining with food.

I walked out of a rock club one night and almost tripped over a short, thin woman seated on the edge of the curb. She was in her mid-thirties, smoking and drinking, kicked back in five-inch heels. She stretched her legs out into the street with ankles crossed as she leaned back on her arms, blowing smoke up into the sky. We made small talk while I shifted around like a teenager in Converse, tugging at my jeans. She exuded ease-of-being in a disarming, nonaggressive way.

Jasmine came from a small town in rural Georgia. Her daddy was an accountant, and Momma stayed home. She out-performed every expectation they had of her professionally but under-performed personally.

She had no interest in having a husband and even less in kids. We spent hours together that night before she confessed to being an attorney, and it wasn't until much later that I found out from other sources exactly how accomplished she was.

She doesn't like being pigeonholed. People assume lawyers are hard, combative, buttoned-up, and unimaginative. She would much rather be known by the hobby she keeps on the side as a massage therapist and reiki practitioner. She's a sucker for a conversation about holistic medicine.

At first, I assumed she didn't care for the law, that it was purely a moneymaker for her, but I couldn't have been more wrong. By the time we met, she was one of the leading legal minds in her field. She loves a challenge. She pursues groundbreaking cases, and almost always wins—but when closing arguments are done, so is she. Her living room is strewn with research files and wool suits, stripped off and left in piles just over the threshold of her front door. She has a Great Dane who shadows her every move. After dark, she can almost always be found on her patio in a cotton maxi-dress, writing firebrand poetry with a cigarette and a mug of red wine.

Her boyfriend is a Chilean surf instructor who travels the world leading month-long surfing retreats, which she attends on a regular basis. They both take lovers on the side, never threatening the foundation of the relationship. They rotate on the same axis, spinning off before circling back and around again. In her words, "I love him precisely because he doesn't bust my balls, and he loves me for the same. Nothing is permanent anyway. He's not mine to keep forever."

She lives that doctrine for the most part but loves him passionately and is not above occasional spirals of jealous online stalking, which bring on painful doubts about her body, clarity of mind, and worthiness. But each time she finds herself in one of those spirals, she finds her center by taking care of her physical body. She throws herself into food and exercise that grounds her. After a while, she remembers that the life she has chosen is the one she wants and settles back into her customary resilience.

Jasmine's job allows her two months of vacation every year, and with that time, there is not a corner of Asia, Africa, Europe, or South America she hasn't seen. She has plenty of money and earned every cent on her own merits. She's five foot three and slim, with an impressive collection of wigs, onesies, and scuffed cowboy boots.

Standing on the street that night, I wanted to write her off. She is one of those little, movie-star-sized people, and I was tempted to hate her out of sheer jealousy. But my experience, training women of all sizes, has taught me that nobody is immune to awkwardness and discontent when dealing with their bodies, and setting up comparisons is pointless. I reluctantly recognized that judging her for being thin would have been as inappropriate and ridiculous as judging her for being heavy. I let her in, and I'm glad I did because, if I had shut her out, I would have deprived myself of one of the greatest friendships of my life.

My weak attempt to pigeonhole her persisted all of twenty seconds before it became clear that she had no interest in being impressive or cute. She wanted to talk about the band and buy me a cocktail. She wanted to lie down on the concrete and identify constellations through the city lights. She wanted to know if I thought people can change, really, truly change, and if so, how?

She is a force of nature, scouring the town in velvet bellbottoms, immersing herself in beautiful music and the musicians that make it— but that's only half of her story.

Jasmine recharges in solitude, sometimes for as long as a month. When she wraps up a case or returns from a long trip overseas, she retreats into extended periods of radio silence. If anyone attempts to break through that silence, he or she is greeted with a dull thud. When she's wrung out, she makes no effort to show up just to be polite. She contributes more to a gathering by staying away when she knows she has nothing to offer. She is uniquely in tune with her body and knows when it needs to rest.

She leaves her front door unlocked year-round so friends can come by to use the house for clandestine work or pleasure whenever necessary, but if they show up during one of her fallow periods, they get nothing out of her but a muffled mumble from an upstairs bedroom. They can have the run of the place. She doesn't mind, but from Jasmine, in her self-imposed isolation, they will get nothing at all. In those weeks or months, she's an attorney and yogi only. She works and sleeps and breathes until she's ready to engage again.

I never know when the hibernation will end, but eventually she emerges. She shows up at my door in flip-flops with a bottle of wine in one hand and a map of the human genome in the other, eager for another night of mind-bending. I've learned to hold space for her when she goes incommunicado because inevitably, out of the silence comes a burst of connectivity—and if I'm lucky, an invitation to a seventies soul dance class and cocktail hour.

She rides instability like rapids on a rafting trip. Instead of exhausting herself by swimming against the tide, she goes for the ride to see where it leads and finds herself deposited on the shore—helmet still strapped on, flotation device intact. She might not have a clue where she landed. She might rest on her back in the sand for a while, but she knows she's on solid ground. She stands up, gets her bearings, and begins moving in whichever direction feels right.

Jasmine has mastered the art of the freefall. When she feels stuck, she uses whatever force is necessary to pry herself loose and then waits, keeping vigil for what follows. She perceives her life as bottomless, openly, almost violently recognizing that much of it is not under her control. She's never sure what's next but has learned, in high style, to live with not knowing. She hasn't always been well-paid and free-wheeling, but she has always been profoundly uncomfortable with paralysis.

Responsible grown-ups might accuse her of being fly-by-night, irresponsible, even selfish, but attorney Jasmine would beg to differ. She is generous with both her time and money. She impacts her community, shaping law and building consensus, and when I ended up in the hospital in the middle of the night a few years ago, she was the one who showed up to hold my hand. She's there without question for the people she loves.

We should all be so lucky to have plenty of time and money and an international love affair to keep things interesting. A life like hers is out of reach for most of us, but I'm not sure I would want it even if I could have it. She may have money, but her life is the furthest thing from secure. Thrill-seeking at that level isn't in the cards for most of us, but her mantra, coined by the writer Neale Donald Walsch, could do us all some good. "Life begins at the end of your comfort zone."[2]

She teaches me how to breathe through my own powerlessness, how to roll around in it and learn from it instead of trying to control it. She teaches me to respect my instincts and the whims of my body, to pull back when something doesn't feel right, and to unapologetically take time alone when the world starts spinning a little too fast.

There are dozens of other women I could offer as examples of how to live courageously and at ease in their bodies; and their stories don't necessarily have anything to do with being footloose or free of responsibility. In fact, the people on planet earth who understand more than anyone else what it means to live well with powerlessness are mothers.

When mothers have done everything they can to support their kids, they understand that their only viable option is to throw their hands up and hope for the best. If they try to hang on and control what the world brings to their kids or what their kids bring to the world, they will drive themselves bat-shit-crazy.

I could dedicate many chapters to the moms who have boggled my mind with their willingness to let go. They are mothers of air force pilots, rock climbers, toddlers with cancer, and tweens in miniskirts. These intrepid women also have aging parents, facing everything from debilitating mental illness to multiple sclerosis. They know powerlessness. They know life's a freefall anyway, so they do every last thing they can to cushion the fall—and then wait to find out whether they'll be cheering from the sidelines or picking up the pieces.

I take my greatest inspiration from this group. I can appreciate the spirited leaps that Sophia and Jasmine take, but I crave structure and balance by nature. In an effort to coax myself and my clients out of cozy but damaging behavior patterns, I've taken a page out of the moms' playbook and found a way to combine structure and release.

I have developed a pod-like approach to my own wellness and taught my clients to do the same. The key is to build a steely infrastructure, an endoskeleton of reliable, fallback behavior and pad the exterior with cotton balls and rubber. To finish, wrap it all up in a triple layer of silver duct tape, and let her roll.

The endoskeleton is made up of solid habits that I know for a fact will keep me sane and healthy; the cotton balls and rubber are open-heartedness and adventure; and the duct tape is the bling, the family and friendships that hold it all together. Inside my pod, I can kick back, knowing that I will fall, bounce, and recover every time.

Part 2 of this book, beginning with the next chapter, is about figuring out specifically what throws you off and what kind of pod you can build to catch the fall.

We are all essentially groundless. The world can drop out from under us at any time. If we can build key systems into our lives—day-to-day habits that strengthen us and set us alight—when the world does drop out: (1) We are not blindsided; (2) We can allow it to hurt and are able to endure whatever pain is necessary; (3) We can turn back to the tangible, predetermined habits we know will hold us up and support our well-being.

In times of crisis, people instinctually get down to basics: arrive at the funeral on time; figure out how to get everybody fed; go to sleep and get up in the morning.

But when there is no crisis, when we're just plain out of shape and annoyed about it, it's a mad dash to get the upper hand. We make rules about eating and proclamations about exercise. We wrestle for con-trol—and fail. Try and fail and try and fail.

What if, instead of going on the attack, we get down to basics? What if we figure out some stuff we like to do that makes us at least a little healthier and don't stop doing it, no matter what annoying, horrible complication arises. There is way too much scheming and planning going on in the fitness universe. There should be more doing.

The crap in our heads is far too muddled. I, for one, was getting nowhere trying to conquer it, so I decided to leave all that clutter alone and turn my focus to my feet—putting one in front of the other on the ground, and not stopping. Ever. I tried things. If one didn't work, I tried something else until I figured out what did. I discovered that I could heal my heart and mind by healing my body first. Not the other way around.

Take a walk. Take a bath. Stretch. Eat an orange. It all starts there.

I only lost a tiny amount of weight at first—maybe a pound a month—but I was getting stronger. The muscles in my legs and arms grew powerful. My lungs reached deeper, and slowly but surely the strength crept into my head. Small changes happened on their own. Cravings began to fade and weaken. The desire to leave parties so I could stop for French fries on the way home started to disappear. My body was gaining ground on my mind.

Whether life is feeling crappy or mighty fine, the same reliable, productive habits will make it better. Figure out what yours are. Keep moving. Keep breathing. Eat something fresh. Over and over. Always the same. Solid ground underfoot. With that in place, a cupcake now and then can be a wonderful way to lift your spirits, a contribution for your body, not a threat.

Taking care of yourself should never be drudgery. If anything, it's an act of defiance. The desire to control your body or subjugate your appearance to somebody else's definition of beauty is destructive. Defy it. Treat your body with reverence and respect. Give it the gift of stepping outside of your comfort zone. Make a practice of loosening your grip, and when you don't know what else to do, coast, and wait for clarity.

Look for the Sophias, Jasmines, and Mignons in your life, the soul shine people. Find them on the news and in the pages of your favorite novels. Breathe them in. Carry them around in your heart, and let them lead you to new and unexpected glimpses of shimmering, clear, blue sky. If these things are constant, you will always be moving toward better and away from worse.

> "The free soul is rare, but you know it when you see it—basically be-
> cause you feel good, very good, when you are near or with them."
> —Charles Bukowski

TOOLBOX

Find your idols.
Remember how you idolized musicians, athletes, or actors as a teenager and strove to be just like them? Find new idols worth emulating, and this time let it be for their fierce dedication to a cause (Alice Walker, author/activist), their willingness to be real (Amy Schumer, comedian, or Lena Dunham, actor/producer/activist), or their ability to roll with the punches without letting it bring them down (Malala Yousafzai, the young, Pakistani, female education advocate who was gunned down by the Taliban but survived and went on to win the Nobel Peace Prize).

Scan your memory banks for people you know personally who have illuminated your life by simply being who they are. Who do you know who is reaching out, refusing to be stymied? Who is actively making peace with her body or stretching beyond her boundaries? They can be friends, family members, mentors, educators, fictional characters, celebrities, or even strangers who set an unintentional example. Write letters to them—which may or may not ever be sent—about how they have ripped the world wide open for you in the most beautiful ways. Embarrass yourself with how much you love and admire them.

Place images of the people and causes that light you up prominently in your space.
Put them on your refrigerator, laptop, bathroom mirror, or phone as reminders (whenever needed) to give your critical inner-monologue a rest, to keep moving forward and opening up to unexplored possibilities. Let them grin their way into your subconscious so that when a

hard day or a series of bad decisions is plaguing you, they can remind you to loosen your grip, reengage, and go along for the ride to see what's next.

How might your role models handle seeing a number on the scale in the morning that they don't like? How might they deal with a traffic jam at the end of a long day? What might they do when feeling beat down other than turn to food? Let them lead the way to a different approach.

Relinquish control of something.

What are you trying to control that you can't? There's always something. What are you trying to hang on to that is taking a toll on your body?

Are you stressed out about your husband's incorrect placement of dishes in the dishwasher? Does it make you want to throw things at his head? Wash your hands of it. Put him 100 percent in charge of it, and never look at it again. If plates break, they break.

Are you freaked out about your three-year-old son's desire to wear a tutu to preschool? Worried what people might think? Buy him a hot pink one and let him twirl.

Are you beating yourself up for having a glass of wine with dinner every night because you're worried about the calories? Don't. Just don't. Wine is good for you.[3] The researchers say so. Let it go.

If you are stress eating or losing sleep due to minor (or even major) issues in your life, figure out what you can let go. Choose at least one small thing to relinquish, and let the cards fall where they may. Odds are everything will turn out fine or, at worst, just the way it would have turned out whether you were fretting over it or not.

Part II

Making It Happen

You turn it on. You turn it off.
And one day you wake to find
you've become the thing
you wished into existence.

—Nick Cave, *20,000 Days on Earth*, 2014

5

HELP YOUR BRAIN HELP YOU

How annoying would it be if I told you that you have ultimate control over the decisions you make and that losing weight and getting healthier is simply a matter of making better ones?

A nutrition professor I had at UCLA told me just that, and I was beyond annoyed—I was pissed. Who did she think she was? Clearly she had no idea how hard I was trying to make better decisions. The situation felt completely out of my control.

Ultimately, I understood that she was right. My choices were my own, but making healthy ones was nowhere near that simple. I felt like a relatively smart, functional person but couldn't wrangle myself into cooperating for longer than a couple of days at a time. My twenty-two-year-old body was puffy and sluggish, and I was driving myself nuts trying to make it better. The Cheerleader was in the ring, throwing punches, but Lothario took her down every time, straight to her back.

I griped over the professor's claim for a few days before realizing that she might be offering a glimpse of blue sky. Maybe, in her overly intellectual, disconnected way, she was offering me a way out. Maybe there was hard science available that could explain why I was having such a difficult time breaking the pattern. Maybe, if I was making the same crappy choices over and over again, someday, with more information or tools at my disposal, I could make different ones—better ones, over and over again.

I felt hostage to a repetitive, unconscious, overwhelming urge to dose myself with sugar and salt, but as I learned more, I discovered that I already possessed the tools needed to interrupt and alter that urge. Within the confines of my own brain, I had everything I needed to begin breaking free of bad habits.

I discovered that one part of my brain is primarily responsible for causing cravings and creating habits, while another determines whether I give in to them and strives for something better. These two brain functions correlate directly with Lothario and the Cheerleader. Once I understood what was happening and how to use each part in the way it was intended, instead of browbeating myself into compliance, I had something tangible to work with.

As human beings, we have the ability to literally, physiologically reshape our brains. It's called neuroplasticity, and it's the coolest science around. It has shown that what you do and the way you think can change the physical structure of your brain. If you repeat a thought pattern or activity enough times in a way that makes your brain feel happy and rewarded, your brain will begin to carve out new neural pathways, and you'll begin to *seek that behavior out*. You'll crave the new activity, and carrying it out will be the path of least resistance.

In other words, your brain isn't stuck the way it is. If your intentions are good but you have zero impulse control, it's not an innate weakness or a failure of willpower. It's not your *fault* on a conscious level. It's the result of natural, evolutionary phenomena buried deep in your gray matter, and with a little key knowledge, it's absolutely within your power to do something about it. There's no reason you have to fight the same old battles for the rest of your life.

The impulsive decisions you make, the ones that feel out of your control, can be changed. The neurological pathways in your brain can be strengthened or weakened depending on which stimuli you give them, and if you give your brain enough good reasons to go after healthy habits, it will continue to look for more opportunities on its own. You can change the urges that rule you by changing your external circumstances.

How strange and amazing would it be if you craved biking more than couch-surfing or beet salad more than pizza?

In the wise words of Dr. Julie Price, PsyD, a licensed clinical health psychologist at Vanderbilt's Osher Center for Integrative Medicine, "It's like a cow path. Cows walk in the same path until they create a rut. That's what happens in your brain. Your nerves go down the same path over and over and create a rut. It's hard coming up and out of it, but you *can* create a new path. It's a slow process, but it definitely can be done."[1]

The bad news is that it's not easy to change. But you knew that already. The good news is that if the cows in your brain lumber down a different path for long enough, that path will become your new, preferred, cozy rut—and if the new rut is a healthy one, that can do a whole lot of good.

A ton of information on this science is available. In the past, researchers believed that after early childhood our brains were fixed and unchangeable—but studies on everything from traumatic brain injury to addiction, meditation to learning disabilities have shown that our brains adapt to what we throw at them.[2]

"The body is an amazing organism, and the brain is no different," says Dr. Price. "It's like a heart or a muscle. We know that the more we use it, the more we stimulate it . . . the more connections are going to grow."

We are physiologically pliable. We have a built-in capacity to change, and once that new behavior becomes a habit, it's not a struggle anymore. It becomes second nature.

Any habit you have, good or bad, exists because at some point you got a quick and easy benefit from it. You drink coffee for the boost. You take city streets at rush hour instead of the freeway because it's faster. You get relief at the end of a stressful day with a movie and a beer. All habits provide a short-term benefit; they only become "bad" habits when they become compulsive or excessive, doing damage in the long run.

There is always a trigger, something that sets you off. For example, you're stressed out about a relationship (or the lack thereof) so you eat to feel better. Eating puts you at ease for a minute before leading to feelings of inadequacy and failure. In that moment of discomfort, you turn back to the original coping mechanism to feel better again—food—which leads to stress leads to food leads to stress. Round and round. The habit itself causes anxiety and begins to perpetuate a cycle of dependence.

Your brain is reaching for bad habits to keep you calm and satisfied. It wants relief as quickly as possible with no regard for the long-term consequences. The impulse to indulge in a destructive habit is Lothario at work, in hot pursuit of immediate gratification, quick and dirty. He wants to know what he can do in the next ten minutes to make you feel better. What is the most beneficial, least effortful option at hand to boost your energy or mood? Carbs, of course! Go get sugary carbs! Or drugs, booze, sex, late-night TV, shopping, driving too fast, checking email too often—anything to boost your serotonin levels lickety-split.

Lothario lives in a part of your brain called the basal ganglia. This is where hardwired information is stored, information you never, ever want to lose: how to brush your hair, ride a bike, or drive a car. These are automated behaviors that you do so well and so often that you don't even know you're doing them half the time. You will never forget how to complete these tasks. They're learned, triggered, and released when they are deemed necessary by a mischievous little monster, buried deep inside the basal ganglia, called the nucleus accumbens.

Every one of your habits, good or bad, is housed and triggered in this part of the brain. Might as well get comfy with them because they will never be forgotten. This is helpful when remembering how to type on your phone. Not so helpful when an oversized muffin and a caramel latte become the only reasonable way to start your morning.

Lothario is rock solid, impulsive, and stubborn. He sees an opportunity for a quick fix and jumps on it. He sees the candy bowl—"CANDY

= HAPPY!" Grab and dash. The habit is released, and it's done before you know what happened.

However, this permanent memory bank has an upside too. It's never full. It's never maxed out. It never runs out of space to store *new* behavior. If given the chance, fresh, healthy habits are perfectly capable of becoming stronger and more reliable, crowding out the nasty, old ones. New ruts can get deeper and wider as older ones lay fallow, overrun by dust and weeds.

The Cheerleader is the prefrontal cortex: thoughtful, reasonable, graceful, and slow. She is seated in your conscious mind. She requires time and attention for analysis and decision making. She allows you to concentrate, plan ahead, and think conceptually. The conscious mind is an elegant thing, but it is notoriously bad at regulating harmful habits. While the Cheerleader is deliberating over what to cook for dinner, Lothario has already driven you to La Hacienda Taqueria for smothered enchiladas and a pitcher of margaritas.

The Cheerleader will never be able to negate engrained, immovable habits. She can't hold them off or beat them back. They can't be erased, *but they can be replaced*. Though she can't get rid of them, she can impact which ones you fall back on and which are expressed on a regular basis.

But how?! If detrimental paths are so well-worn, how exactly can you hope to create new ones? You might assume that willpower is at the center of any change like this, and in a way, you're right, but odds are you are trying to use it in exactly the wrong way. Willpower does make change possible but not in the way we traditionally think.

Willpower is essentially useless if you are trying to *stop* a behavior. It can help you focus on proactively *doing* something, but if you are trying to *avoid* doing something—not eating the candy in the candy bowl, for instance—it's basically worthless, especially over the long haul.

Willpower is a conscious process. It originates in the prefrontal cortex and requires placing what you're doing at the center of your mind. If your objective is to *not* do something, focusing on it makes it nearly impossible to resist. If you spend all day telling yourself, "Don't think about the candy bowl!" Of course, all you can think about is the candy bowl.

If you rely on willpower to resist a bad habit, you can be sure it will fail you. The Cheerleader will end up in a sniveling heap on the ground while Lothario coyly unwraps one delicious, mouthwatering chocolate at a time. But if you use willpower to support *new* habits, you've got a good shot. Instead of resisting candy from the candy bowl, use willpower to put a bunch of grapes in a bag—bring them to work, place them on your desk, and eat one every time you think of the candy dish.

Willpower can create systems that will buttress your new choices. It can provide you with healthy options and make them easier to act on. The new choices might feel clumsy and awkward at first, but having a plan in place when old impulses flare up can be a huge relief. That knowledge alone, that you have something specific to turn to, can reduce your stress level and make you less susceptible to bad habits.

When implementing real changes, there is a method to the madness, and that method isn't really all that complicated. The steps themselves are straightforward. I don't mean to imply that they're easy to follow, but they are relatively simple. The hard part is staying mindful of them, and applying them in your life with enough regularity to see results.

In the fleeting moment that you're making a decision about whether to engage in a bad habit, you can make a healthier choice if you can consciously recognize the urge when it first arises—halt the urge before you react—and provide yourself with immediate access to alternatives that bring at least some measure of satisfaction. It's no small task, but the following steps can help.

1. Identify and manage triggers. Figure out what happens just before your bad habit swoops in and takes over. Charles Duhigg's book *The Power of Habit* popularized well-established habit change techniques based in cognitive-behavioral therapy and is a wonderful resource.[3] He outlines five simple, but extremely helpful questions to ask when you're figuring out what triggers a bad habit: (1) Where are you?

(2) What time is it? (3) What is your emotional state? (4) Who else is around? (5)What action preceded the urge?

Watch for that initial impulse. Identify when, where and how it arrives so you can head it off at the pass. Any time you find yourself in the middle of a "bad" habit, jot down the surrounding circumstances in shorthand, and see if you can find a pattern.

Once you've identified when or why it happens, do whatever you can to reduce your exposure to the triggers. Stress comes from every-where—lack of sleep, a bad phone call, an unhealthy work environ-ment, the evening news, loneliness, financial strain, relationships, con-cern over people you love. Some triggers are certainly beyond your control, but do what you can to limit stressors anywhere and every-where you do have control. It can be something as small as seeing a sign for your favorite restaurant on your way home from work. Take a differ-ent route.

2. Reframe old habits. Create new associations for bad habits. You know how you feel about a meal that has recently given you food poi-soning? The thought of it turns your stomach in the weeks immediately following the exposure. No matter how much you loved the food be-fore, you suddenly have no desire to eat it again. That is a new, learned association. Pad Thai equals vomiting. Gross!

Actively associate your old habits with feeling terrible. Food poison-ing is a bit drastic, but the connections are there if you look for them. Fast food equals bloating. An entire box of cookies before bed equals a restless night and a pinched waistline in the morning meeting. Overex-erting yourself at the gym or not taking the time to learn proper form equals knee pain. Purposefully make new, negative associations with old habits. Stamp a word on them. Label them with something that reflex-ively turns you off, and recall that word when the habit pops up. Don't place judgment on it; just build in a new cause and effect. French fries equal zits.

3. Choose a competing habit. Select at least one (or preferably a few) specific, alternate, and desirable habits that you can turn to in place of the thing you don't want to do anymore. When your boss is a jerk, instead of heading for the vending machine, go for a walk around the building. When *this* happens [insert stressor], I will do *that* [insert new habit].

When this, then that. Make the new habit something you truly enjoy while you're in the middle of it, at least a little bit.

4. Preplan. Have a system in place to make the new habit as easy and accessible as possible. Do everything you can to make the new choice a no-brainer. Put sneakers under your desk. Leave your wallet in the glove compartment so you don't have cash for unplanned snacks. Keep a giant bowl of prewashed fruit on the kitchen counter. When the urge for the old thing arises, close your eyes, take a deep breath, and consider your options.

5. Repeat without judgment. When you do fall back on the old habit, don't be surprised. It's part of the deal. That's how this works. The consequences of the bad habit are there to remind you again why you don't want to do that anymore—and you'll need *a lot* of reminding before the new habit becomes the easy choice. Notice the impact of the bad habit every time you engage it, register how it feels, and set it aside. Another chance to make a different choice will arrive again very soon, and if you're still beating yourself up from the last time you gave in, you'll be too stressed out to make a better choice.

Watch for triggers. Keep new options at the forefront of your mind, and choose them as often as you can. You may have to offer yourself an alternate habit for weeks before you actually choose it. That's fine. Keep it on the table. If you're never able to make that new choice, try a different alternate or choose a different bad habit to address. Uproot the routine however you can. If you must visit the vending machine, do it, but instead of taking the chips back to your desk, take them out for a stroll instead. Do something, anything, to signal your brain that change is in motion.

Behind each one of these steps is the question of thirst. The whole pursuit will fizzle and fade if it's not for a cause that lights you up. The effort to stay aware, plan ahead, and adjust your perspective requires an enormous amount of brainpower. You'll run out of steam one way or the other, but if you have something you want really, really badly driving the whole thing, you'll be much more likely to get back to it. You'll rest up and try again, and again, until it begins to stick.

The desire, the thirst that drives you, can be perky and proactive. It can be for a good cause if that works for you: to set a good example for somebody else or to feel better in your clothes. If that works, fantastic, but if it doesn't, consider appealing to darker motives.

Your reason for taking care of yourself should be whatever works. If traditional motivators aren't working, toy with being a little competitive, snarky, or fueled by revenge. If that's what's happening in your head anyway, you might as well use it for good. Nobody has to know as long as it's not doing harm to anyone. You don't have to tell a single soul what drives you, but it absolutely has to be something that strikes a chord. When you pause and bring it to mind at the center of a choice between candy and grapes, your thirst for the big picture should outweigh your desire for candy. The system will be in place, the options will be before you, and thirst will serve as a final push needed to make the better choice.

Once the changes begin to bear fruit—a leaner body, greater confidence, or decreasing aches and pains—the driving force behind it can and should begin to shift away from negative reinforcements, toward positive pursuit of weightlessness and freedom. But in the meantime, at the beginning, all motives are good ones as long as they fire you up and don't hurt anybody else in the process.

Allow me to offer a real-life example—a twisted one, but sometimes those are the best kind. In my mid-twenties, I dated a guy named Antonio. He was a bachelor to the bitter end, twelve years older than me, tall, dark, Italian, blue-eyed, wealthy, and foul. He taught me about fancy cheese and Spanish wine. Food was a celebration for him, and exercise a religion.

He lavished affection on me but downplayed our relationship to his friends and family. He never wanted to leave the house except in search of food or films that could be brought back to our enclave. He would disappear for weeks at a time under the guise of working too much, only making himself available in the dead of the night, and then whisk me away on breathtaking, erotic weekends to San Francisco or Zion National Park. He held me at bay most of the time and lured me back in when I began to drift. Together, we were volatile, electric, and utterly defective.

The situation was far from healthy. It was a maze of infatuation and frustration, but I began to draw a perverted sort of strength from Antonio's unavailability. In forced solitude, enduring weeks of intermittent calls, body heat followed by the chill of silence, I set out to prove that I was worthy of his lasting affection. In the past, that kind of unrelenting rejection would have sent me further into lethargy and food addiction, but this particular relationship was too deeply rooted in a physical bond. Letting my body go would have been equivalent to letting *him* go, not because he would have judged me—all flesh was good flesh to him— but because I would have been less alive in my skin. The greater my connection with my own body, the greater my connection with his. The desire to dive deeper with him propelled me to the gym with rabid devotion.

Living in the shadows of Antonio's life, I took every bit of anger and resentment I had for him straight to the treadmill and weight bench. I memorized exercise routines like Bible verses and followed them to the letter of the law. I was steeped in wicked, agonizing lust, and it drove me to take care of myself with a force I had never imagined possible. What I didn't anticipate was that as my body got stronger, so would my mind.

What began as a way of showing Antonio that I was good enough to win his love ended up irrevocably changing my body and the structure of my brain. It gave me the strength to leave him behind once and for all. Two years after we met, I stood on a sidewalk in West Hollywood, spitting words at him with fingernails flashing, my teeth on edge, finally powerful enough—body and mind—to walk away. My motivation from the very beginning was questionable. I was parched for his affection.

That thirst may have been misguided, but it was honest. It propelled me forward until I began to notice changes rising up from underneath.

Fortunately, exercise works no matter the motivation, and I came out of those two years with no doubt about the effect strength training could have on my brain, mood, and confidence. It was a powerful lesson I could never unlearn, and by the time it was over, I had new, unforeseen, healthy coping mechanisms in place that I could continue building on for the rest of my life. They were motivated initially by lust, but maintained because they made me better, more myself.

Lothario still showed up on lonely Saturday nights to serve up a pint of ice cream, but the resulting guilt wasn't there anymore. I let my messy, old habits be there. They were too hard to change and brought too much vital comfort. Many of them persisted for years to come, but they were steadily encroached upon, crowded out by a growing notion of what it felt like to be light on my feet, strong, and validated—with or without Antonio.

I had no conscious awareness of how I was motivating myself until it was done. I had no idea that I was implementing scientifically sound behavioral modification techniques. I went after something I wanted very badly and didn't end up getting it. The whole pursuit could have been seen as a failure if I hadn't gained something so much more valuable.

My body and mind changed because I pursued what I wanted using methods that *enriched my life*. I allocated my energy doing something good instead of trying to prevent something bad and ended up so much better off, with a long list of options, steps to take, and things to do when stress and anxiety began building again.

As I walked away from Antonio, down the sidewalk in West Hollywood with my heart on the pavement behind me, groundless again, I had something new holding me up. I was physically well, and that wellness made everything better. From then on, whenever that sensation began to slip away, I thirsted for it and sought it out using the steps I had learned so well, turning back to them for support. The sensation of wellness itself became the new motivation, and it was mine to access no matter what else was happening in my life.

At the beginning and in the middle of trying to change, the effort didn't feel transformative. It felt like moving through mud. At first, Antonio was both the trigger and the thirst. He set me on a destructive path and fired me up to pursue well-being at the same time. The forces behind my new habits might have been dubious, but the habits themselves took over in the end, molding my body into an instrument that served *me*, not him.

Behavioral patterns are within your control if you are willing to put sustained, conscious, unemotional effort into changing them. Your brain is in search of relief—that's all. Put the Cheerleader in charge of finding new ways to get that relief, and lean on the steps above to forge a pristine, new rut—one you can get comfy in, one that leads directly to your old lady, your Malibu hillside, and your paintbrush.

TOOLBOX

Pick one specific (but small) habit to change and replace it with another. Consider this a practice run. Choose something that won't be too difficult to tweak.

1. *Identify and manage your triggers.* When and why does it happen, and how can you avoid exposure to those circumstances?
2. *Reframe old habits.* Associate the bad habit with grossness. Skipping your walk equals foggy brain or depression. Bacon cheeseburger equals constipation. Recall the association whenever the negative impulse comes up.
3. *Choose a competing habit.* Something you like. When this urge comes up, I will do that. When this, then that.
4. *Preplan.* Supply every reinforcement possible to make the new choice easier. Prepack the gym bag and put it in the car. Stock

your fridge or desk with precut or precooked fruits and veggies you can snack on all day.

5. *Repeat without judgment.* It doesn't matter if you "fail" to make the healthy choice at first. Don't beat yourself up. Keep reminding yourself that the new thing is there if you want it. *It's there if I want it. It's there if I want it. Oh yeah! It's there! I think I'll try it!* If, eventually, it looks like the change you picked is not ever going to happen, shoot for a different one. No biggie. Just keep moving, keep trying this or that until something works.

Dig up whatever thirst works.

Try different motivations on for size, and get subversive if need be. Secretly compete with somebody in your head, or do it to prove to your boss that you won't let her daily stress-party take you down. It doesn't have to be pretty, at least not at the beginning. Or try a more positive motivator. Be a role model for your partner or kids, or do it for your health, to reduce pain or the onset of disease. Set up a contest with your friends with a cool prize at the end. If the thing you thought would work isn't successfully driving you, try something else and keep looking until something gets you moving.

6

STRENGTH OUTSIDE IN

A client named Paul taught me everything I could ever hope to know about how to make change stick. He confirmed a sneaking suspicion I had in my early years as a trainer that bodies and lives are most easily transformed from the outside in.

We don't always have to deconstruct the causes of bad habits before we can move forward. Instead of spending months and years trying to dig through vague and unwieldy psychodrama, sometimes it's easier to focus on the tangible actions of feet and hands. Concrete changes are manageable and can create space for the psychological stuff to work itself out. New habits can be introduced and documented, and if chosen specifically because they enrich your life, they don't have to be all that difficult to maintain.

Paul changed his life by focusing on what could be done in the present. He built new and different rituals into his days that signaled his brain that change was happening. He pounded out different paths—fresh, healthy ruts—that will continue to serve him for the rest of his life.

I met Paul on a January evening in the lounge on the top floor of the high-rise building where he lived. He was in his mid-fifties with stooped posture, a rounded belly, and dark circles under his eyes. His hair was combed properly to the side, his hands folded in his lap as he sat hunched over on the couch. His father had recently passed away. He was twice divorced with a daughter in college. The second marriage lasted only a few months and left him reeling when it ended.

He held the same middle management job for decades. His work was suffering from all of the changes in his personal life, but his boss and coworkers were flexible and supportive of his need to take care of himself, to take time for appointments with doctors, psychologists, and now, a personal trainer.

He had palpable anxiety and a great deal of difficulty focusing. During that first conversation in the lounge, his attention wandered. I had to repeat questions several times, forcefully searching for answers as he checked out of our discussion and drifted off to wherever his thoughts were calling him. At times, he didn't appear to register that I was speaking to him at all as he stared down at the floor, chin almost resting on his chest, eyes averted, and shoulders slumped.

He could see clearly, and expressed concisely, the hole he was sitting in, the dustiness of a body unmoved and a heart misjudged. But he was actively engaging the world on multiple fronts: psychotherapy, exercise, wine tastings, gallery openings, and hockey games. He was reaching for any hand that could help him climb a few inches farther out of the ditch.

I was impressed. He was bruised and beaten but not going down without a fight. With gray hair and a rumpled suit, he had a fire to be greater and more fulfilled than he currently was. He was on the right path. None of his chosen therapies or activities by themselves would be likely to result in long-term healing, but all of them together gave him a very good shot.

We started slowly, testing his limits and endurance. Much to my surprise, and his own, he proved to be an easy athlete. He was swift on the treadmill, and his heart could support significant challenges without exhausting him. He gained strength quickly and started dropping weight. He didn't have all that much to lose, maybe twenty pounds, but as his face slimmed down, his skin began to brighten. He sat up straighter and began cracking jokes during our sessions. We discovered we had a lot in common and a compatible sense of humor. He set aside a lifelong aversion to sweating and arrived at our scheduled appointments with spectacular consistency. He was *never* late. He never missed a session without giving me plenty of notice, and that only happened in the most extreme circumstances.

Often, when I first start working with people who are juggling multiple issues—especially those hovering at the edge of depression—there are lots of cancellations. Their minds trick them into believing that they have insurmountable obstacles, aches and pains, injuries, scheduling conflicts and overall exhaustion. I'm sure every one of those excuses passed through Paul's mind, but he was stoic, stubborn. He put his head down and plowed ahead. He showed up no matter what. During most sessions, I had to repeat myself three or four times before he paid attention to which exercise was next, but once he snapped to and heard my instructions, he was off and running, completing the sets with precision.

Some days were tougher than others. His eyes would retreat into their sockets, his chest caving in under the pressure of a brother struggling with chronic illness and a mother widowed. His first wife was remarried, and his daughter was focused on school. He had good friends but was often alone in his bachelor pad on the eighteenth floor.

With floor to ceiling windows, he could look out over the city at night, buzzing with tourists wandering in and out of nightclubs and locals lugging guitar cases up and down the steep streets leading to Lower Broadway. His mind wandered and energy waned, but in our sessions, his body was always present and accounted for.

Years of stress had weakened his upper back, shortening and binding his chest, creating a stooped silhouette and aging him long before his time. On hard days when he seemed particularly weighed down, I had him lie down on his back on the floor, stretching his arms up over his head as far as they could reach. I pressed down slowly on his palms until the backs of his hands could touch the floor. His stress had found a protective home in his pectoral (chest) muscles, safely tucking itself away under sinewy, stiff musculature and taut, inflexible shoulder joints—and his relief at opening that space was visible.

Much of our work was about opening this area of his body and strengthening weakened rhomboids, lats, and rear deltoids—the muscles in his upper back that could help him stand up straight. We stretched his chest, strengthened, and stretched again.

I began to see a new man showing up for our sessions: taller, slimmer, flashing fire a lot closer to the surface. He started dating again and bought a motorcycle. He was transforming before my eyes. His sense of well-being and vitality seemed in direct proportion with his commitment to fitness, and watching him step out of the shadows remains one of the most rewarding experiences of my career.

Paul's willingness to try new things gave him access to a world of possibilities, but what made the greatest difference over time, through good days and bad, was consistency. He did not allow himself to shrink back into his old life. He showed up, no matter what. Sluggish or energized, he was there—and over time, that steady commitment changed the structure of his days, the rhythm of his nights, and the nature of his mind.

Paul's health was improving rapidly, along with his state of mind. He was making enormous strides in strength and flexibility when he got hit with a series of obstacles that could have stymied pretty much anyone.

He had a motorcycle accident that left him with two badly sprained ankles and cuts and bruises all over his body. Most of the injuries healed within a few weeks, but one of the ankles persisted and remained painful for months. We adjusted his program, keeping him moving without irritating the injury. He pushed through, always willing to do whatever he could.

After that, he discovered bone spurs growing in his right shoulder and knee. He underwent surgery to remove them, but a full recovery to pain-free status took many months longer than the doctors anticipated. As he waited for the pain to subside, we pressed on, gently strengthening the joints, working around them and bringing them back.

Nothing threw him. He was unyielding in his devotion to the everyday changes that had made him feel so much better. There was no magic at work here, and he knew it. His health sat at the center of everything else in his life, and he chose to maintain it in any and every way possible, even as one challenge after another arose.

As he began to feel better, he ventured into the world of online dating. After a few ill-fitting, short-term relationships, Paul told me softly about a woman he met named Eliza. She was a guidance counselor in a public high school and an artist on her own time. She was divorced with grown kids, trying to get back on her feet after an abusive, unhealthy marriage. Eliza was tall and lanky, beautiful and earthy. She cherished Paul for the gentle, thoughtful man he was, and within months, she moved in with him.

She came home one day with a tiny, little man she had made of white clay. He was about three inches tall, sitting on his heels with his legs folded under him. His hands were clasped in his lap like a little kid, face wide and round but wrinkled with age, posture bowed over like an old man. His head was cocked with eyes turned to the sky and a huge Buddha-like grin on his face. He was playful, sad, and spiritual all at the same time. I reached out to touch him and was warned that he was made of soft clay like silly putty; he would never harden and dry. We simply had to let him be, which made her creation even sweeter. This little man was fragile. He was malleable, open-hearted, and beautiful.

He reminded me of Paul and, frankly, of all of my other clients—and even me. When we are able to be wide-eyed and childlike, halfway broken and halfway healed at the same time, and to continue looking up and out for joyfulness, it's a remarkable thing to behold. That openness affords us enormous potential for growth, and I've been blessed to see it happen in people of every shape and size, at every phase of weight loss or gain.

Eliza continued bringing in pieces of art she created in drawing and painting workshops. Paul continued to fall in love with her, and I continued to fall in love with her art and the idea of the two of them together. They made each other better, more stable, happier, and stronger. They got engaged, and soon after that, Eliza's mother passed away. Paul stood by her, supporting her however she needed and treating her grown children like his own.

The biggest hit Paul took was when a routine stress test on his heart came back abnormal. He had an arrhythmia. As he put it, the problem was with the electrical, not the plumbing. This sent him back to the hospital yet again, this time for an arteriogram and an invasive procedure called ablation to mitigate his racing heart. After almost a week in the hospital, bruised and sore from shots and tubes, he was released, but the heart medications made him dizzy and weak.

Two days after he got home, we were scheduled to meet for a workout. He called in the afternoon saying that he had a dizzy spell getting out of his car on his way to work; the side of his groin was purple and aching where they had inserted the catheter to snake their way up to his heart; and his energy was waning—all common side effects for patients who have undergone an arteriogram. I assumed he needed more time to heal, but he was calling to say that he very much wanted me to come that day.

He had been in a hospital bed for too long and felt stiff and bloated from the fluids they pumped into him. He knew exercise would make him feel better but was afraid to do it alone. When I met him in the gym that night, he looked almost as pale and puffy as he did the day we met. We did basic exercises with light weights. He rode for a few minutes on the stationary bike where he could sit and keep his balance, and we stretched, taking back a body that felt invaded. By the end of the hour, he was looser and lighter.

A few weeks later, the bloat was gone. The bruises were reduced to gray halos of their previous shapes, but his new medications made him lethargic until his doctor found the right cocktail of meds. His struggle with an irregular heart rate continued, but he never wavered in his determination to keep moving at whatever pace he could. We closely followed the medical instructions given to him and continued to seek out the safest, best ways to stay in motion—and, of course, Eliza stayed by his side the whole way.

Paul sees gentle, regular exercise as non-negotiable. It heals him. No matter what comes at him, he presses on, determined to take care of the only body he has. He refuses to return to his previous self—a lonely middle manager with a beer belly and an empty apartment in a high-rise building—and sees exercise as a basic component of his overall wellness.

His new life and woman are vibrant and warm. He couldn't have found her and held on to her if he hadn't taken care of himself in the first place. He would never have had the energy to take long bike rides with her or the confidence to create a shelter for her, a peaceful spot to lay her struggles down and start building her own strength in the arms of a man who had come so far in finding peace of mind.

Paul and I took similar paths to extricate ourselves from stagnation and heartbreak. We altered the landscape of our lives from the outside in: building physical strength; finding people and activities that nourished us; and changing basic behavior patterns to effect an inner shift. Sometimes changes came slowly, one at a time, and sometimes they came in clusters.

When I stepped out on the sidewalks of New York City, one foot in front of the other, looking for little bits of clear blue sky, that was all I could manage. I started walking, and that was all. But once I got going, I took a reckless approach, running like a bandit from one city to another, changing jobs, apartments, and men—never looking back. With each change, I lurched forward into a slightly happier existence and a more peaceful relationship with my body.

Paul took a more measured path. He managed to stay in his city, job, and apartment while completely recreating his way of life. When he signed up for therapy, personal training, and wine tasting, he needed them all to happen simultaneously for any of them to seem doable.

Working with Paul confirmed for me what previously I only hoped to be true. Identity does not have to be static; it can move and change with time and place. He made a decision not to be defined by his occupation or divorces. He didn't have to be a lonely businessman. He could be a wine aficionado and a monster hockey fan. He could be a great dad and newly awakened lover. He could be a biker dude on Saturdays if that's what he wanted.

The structure of your life as it is right now supports the body you have right now, and something about that structure will have to be markedly different to support a different one. Your job, your lover, your city, your evenings, your mornings, your friends, your shopping habits—something will have to change, probably several somethings. If not, everything, including your body, will remain the same.

We are all entrenched in something, and that's fine. We need a certain level of comfort and familiarity to make the ride easier. Sometimes the worst habits are the ones most worth hanging on to at the beginning. Knowing they're there at the end of the day to keep you sane can help smooth things over as you tackle smaller ones, but eventually small changes begin to engulf the bigger ones, making them seem less challenging than they once were. You *can* alter your routine without freaking yourself out. It's just a matter of figuring out where to begin. These things tend to have a domino effect, and they don't necessarily need to have anything to do with diet or exercise. Changing your bedtime, mealtimes, or the way you interact with media (television or otherwise) can have far-reaching effects.

Take a look at your top three bad habits. Give serious thought to what it would be like to live without each one. Does it feel like too steep of a climb? Have you tried to quit multiple times and failed? What if you knew for a fact that you had the others to hang on to? Would that make it easier? Inch your way down the list of vices you don't want to live with any more until you find one you think you can tackle, and leave the others alone.

Deliberately choose the "bad" habits that you want to continue, and rely on them whenever you're in need. Claim them as your own. Allow them to be the release valves that they are, free and clear. Cherish them—at least for the time being—because you're probably going to continue engaging in them whether you want to or not, so you might as well enjoy them. Let them be your own personal, beautiful, detrimental choice. Live inside of them; love them; notice them; feel them; hate them; find comfort in them; and repeat them. On and on for as long as you want.

If you know for a fact that you're going to stop beating yourself up for late-night eating, would it make breakfast or afternoon snack choices easier to handle?

The idea is to get stronger and healthier in as many areas of your life as possible, until any remaining habits still causing more harm than good begin to feel like a bad fit. Eventually, the ones that are truly destructive will begin to stick out like a sore thumb, and you'll grow tired of them naturally.

When you have chosen one thing to change, use the five steps from the previous chapter to isolate and replace it. Once the new habit becomes second nature and you've had a taste of success, you can shoot for the next one, maybe something bigger with even greater impact.

All you're doing is replacing one negative with one positive and doing it as consistently as possible. Consistency is crucial—it forges that new, well-worn path in your brain. Of course, you will likely fall back many times on old behavior. It doesn't matter. Just keep moving and coming back to the new habit again and again, forging change from the outside in.

As I said before, the new choice will probably feel forced at first. It will take effort, but it should *always* bring some sort of immediate gratification. It should feel at least a little good, right away.

When this, then that.

When you've already had dinner and half of an oversized chocolate bar and you want nothing more than to break out a box of cookies, *do something else* before you dive in. Pick up a guitar. Eat an ice cube. Do ten squats. Take a shower. Eat a banana.

When you're done with that, if a box of cookies still seems like the best course of action, go for it *without apology*. If you're going to do it, go ahead and savor it. Remember that the ultimate goal is freedom, enjoyment of your body and life. Let the cookies taste good while you're

busy filling the rest of the open space in your days with healthy, restora-
tive food and activities. Cookies pose no threat to you. They aren't
illicit. They're just sweet treats. That's all. So let them happen if that's
what you need. Just keep looking around for what else you can do, in
addition, to reinforce your health.

This process is not about denying yourself. It's about interrupting
autopilot and attempting to fill the void with something else first. You're
building new routines to support your own liberty, a steel framework
that will allow you to uphold your health to the best of your ability no
matter what state of mind you're in or what obstacles you encounter.

Miserable or vibrant, you will know without a doubt which habits
keep your head above water and which pull you under. The basics will
keep you afloat. Anything above and beyond that will give you enough
breathing room to let your mind wander to what else might be possible.
Imagination unhinged.

During the six years I lived in L.A., I hiked up into Griffith Park
almost every day. The days I wanted to do it the least were the ones
when I needed it the most. My hamstrings and calves dug into the
hillside as I breathed in daylight and pushed my speed to get above the
smog line where everything was clear. It took forty-five minutes top to
bottom, and without fail, whatever my frame of mind when I left, by the
time I made it to the top, I was better, lighter, and freer.

If coaxed and activated daily, your body will respond and your mind
will follow. Small repetitive actions make an enormous difference over
the course of a lifetime. If whatever is happening inside your head is too
muddled to wade through, let strength come from the outside in, one
tangible habit at a time.

TOOLBOX

Be consistent.

Whatever new habit you're implementing, be persistent about it. Your
brain will forget how good the new habit feels as it tries to lead you back

to the old one. Blindly, stubbornly implement the new one until your brain catches up and realizes what it's been missing out on all along.

Pick your poison.

Actively choose which bad habits you still need, and release yourself from any guilt in association with them. You're going to keep doing them anyway, so you might as well enjoy them.

Do something new and different.

Yes, it can be nerve racking to try something new, but doing something cool and fun and adventurous will pry open your brain to allow for a different relationship with your body and mind. It works like travel. Exposure to new things can't help but stretch your mind.

Do something unfamiliar (or something you haven't done in forever) once a week for a month. Once a week isn't too big of a task. Take a walk at a park you've never been to; take a fitness class you've never tried; go out on a paddleboat on a lake; take a pottery class; go on a blind date; go bowling; play mini-golf; try a new recipe; go horseback riding; invite an acquaintance you'd like to get to know better out for lunch; volunteer to help build a house; offer to walk an elderly neighbor's dog; see what's happening at a local community center; go to one of those giant trampoline places; go swimming with a kickboard; draw a picture; call up a grad school you've been thinking about and have them send you a pamphlet.

The options are endless. Refer back to the list you made in chapter 2 to see what new adventures might be worth thirsting for.

7

DODGING THE YO-YO

A friend of mine named Mark passed away a few years ago. He was thirty-eight years old, an avid runner, a healthy eater, and one of the kindest people I have ever known. His heart stopped in the middle of the night as he lay in bed next to his pregnant wife, with their one-year-old son asleep in the next room. The doctors discovered later that he had some sort of rare, undetectable heart defect, but as far as any of us knew at the time, he was healthy and strong until the day he died.

I was in a habit at the time, of telling my clients that staying healthy is important for longevity, preventing disease, and such, but with his passing, I realized that longevity is only one of many powerful reasons to take good care of ourselves. Staying healthy isn't about the number of days we have on earth. It's about the quality of the days we have while we're here; it's about how we feel in our bodies all day, every day.

If Mark had known that he only had thirty-eight years to live, I doubt he would have done it any differently. I don't think he would have opted out of his daily three-mile run, which made his days feel more alive. Time spent with his son, family, friends, and at work was all informed by the state of his body, and his body was vibrant and at ease.

If exercising and eating well help us live longer, that's wonderful, but what matters even more is how we feel right now. With Mark's passing, my focus on being "thin" took a major body blow. I realized that what was most important was to feel at least okay—and at best exuberant—in the body I was blessed to inhabit. My friend didn't have the luxury of living in his body anymore. I had mine, but I had squandered the previous decade battling it. I wanted to spend however many more days I had nurturing and utilizing it. Another minute spent hating myself for carrying around extra weight was a minute of my life trivialized. The clock was running out on my bullshit. I was beginning to see with greater clarity that beating myself up was a worthless and destructive pastime.

Weight is irrelevant. It's literally just a measurement of the force of gravity on our bodies. Allowing our happiness to be affected by how high or low that force is on any given day is a waste. We can spend our lives worshiping at the altar of weight loss and being haunted by a relentless battle with food, or we can choose to prioritize feeling stronger and moving more freely.

The more I sit with that choice, the more obvious it becomes. It's a no-brainer.

Food has a direct impact on the quality of our lives: energy, sleep, digestion, skin, focus, mood—the list goes on. There are countless cues available to signal to us which food will energize us and which will drag us down, but most of the time we're profoundly out of touch with those cues. We're not paying attention. Life is demanding. It's a lot simpler to make arbitrary rules about what we can and cannot do, and try to follow them, than it is to actually listen to our bodies on a regular basis. But those kinds of rules have no connection to what is feasible, much less what might be enjoyable, on a long-term basis. We try to control and restrict ourselves and end up completely detaching from our bodies in the process.

We isolate a "bad food" (usually one we adore), and quit it. Bread, anyone? We subsist on "energy" bars and wonder why we can't ever get to the gym at the end of the day. We become irrational and sleepy while counting calories and eating bland, boring food—and it's a big, fat bummer, so we give up. Until the next time.

Counting calories is useful only for people who do not understand that ice cream and soda can make you gain weight. I don't say that in jest. Many people lack access to nutritional education or have simply never given much thought to what they're eating. I have had such people as clients, and for them, it's genuinely helpful to see the sad face appear on their food diary app after eating a burger and onion rings for lunch. But for those of us with a basic handle on which foods and methods of preparation are more or less healthy, counting calories takes us further away from perceiving on a visceral level how much is too much and what feels right when a meal is over.

We don't need more control. We need greater awareness of how food actually feels, how stagnation or stimulation physically impact us. You can't get a body you love by doing things that you hate. Even if you manage to lose weight by strong-arming yourself for a few months, there's no pleasure in the outcome. It's unsustainable and tiresome.

Our bodies want to maintain equilibrium. They instinctually strive to sustain balance and good health. When we have a cold, our immune system beats it back. When we break a leg, it heals. The systems of the body work together with incredible synchronicity to keep us functioning at our best, but we're so far out of touch that we can't decide whether we're hungry or just bored. We can't tell if a plate of buffalo wings will make us feel better or worse.

An awareness of what feels good—featherweight good—is the greatest tool you have for building a body that fits. Your brain will trick you into thinking a bagel and cream cheese every morning feels "good," but your body will not. It will feel lighter or heavier, more energized or sluggish depending on how much you move and what you eat. Figuring out the difference is the only way to create changes that will hold up effortlessly for the rest of your life.

I met a woman named Georgia on my doorstep one evening while she was taking a lost dog door to door, looking for his owner. Within about thirty minutes she would become a client, and over the next nine months she would smoke me in the weight loss game, leaving me in the dust. But even faster than she lost it, she would gain it all back. She was disconnected from her body and mind, with no awareness at all of when she felt balanced and when she felt dysfunctional—and that disconnect cost her dearly.

We made small talk on the porch that first night, and when I mentioned that I was a trainer, she launched into an enthusiastic, rapid-fire monologue: *She didn't usually look fat like this; her friends could barely recognize her anymore; and she was much more shy with strangers than she used to be since she gained a whole bunch of weight; and she didn't know what to do; and it must be fate that we met; and now I could be her personal trainer and get her in shape so she could go to a reunion with her college friends and show them how much better she looked; and she couldn't believe her luck that the dog came into to her yard because now everything was going to work out great!*

I get this sort of self-effacing diatribe a lot, but she had them all beat.

I saw no evidence of her supposed shyness. From what I could gather, she was a fourth grade teacher in her early thirties, about 185 pounds, five foot seven with a remarkable amount of energy. She had a lilting southern accent and very little awareness of the normal give and take of polite adult conversation. She had pale skin with long, straight, dark hair down to her waist, a few light brown freckles, and pencil thin arms. She carried all of her weight from the waist down. Georgia loved dogs and told me about the two she had recently adopted—*and her husband and her husband's cousin who lived in L.A. and her family and her house and her job, and anyway, a personal trainer was exactly what she needed!!!*

I nodded, trying to get a word in edgewise, but mostly I just listened as she continued on at warp speed. We set a time to meet for a workout, and I tried to imagine how I might tame her tirades long enough to accomplish anything.

On my first visit, I met her husband who was soft spoken and easygoing. The house was a disaster with piles of children's books, celebrity magazines, and chick-lit novels. Her sneakers were chewed up by the dogs, so that one lace on each shoe only extended about an inch beyond the top hole. Half-eaten rawhides were strewn all over the floor, as well as mutilated yogurt containers given to the dogs for after-dinner treats. She and her husband faithfully tried to maintain some degree of order, but the battle was lost before it began.

Georgia launched into an explanation for the mess, which I reassured her was unnecessary. I wasn't going to judge them for having a messy house. In fact, I appreciated the honesty. Honesty is one of the best predictors of success in my clients. If they are honest with themselves and with me, their chances of making progress are infinitely better.

She set up a spare bedroom for our workout space with a decent treadmill from Goodwill, some hand weights, an ancient stationary bike (circa 1982), a yoga mat, and a balance ball—everything she might need to get in shape. I was worried that she wouldn't be capable of focusing, but my concern couldn't have been more displaced.

She hit the ground running with three, hour-long training sessions per week, each consisting of cardio, weights, and stretching. She joined a popular diet program based on prepackaged food, and planned her snacks each night for the following day.

The exercises she liked best required full-body engagement rather than precise movement of one body part at a time. Though physically more demanding, any exercise that required her to swing or jump with multiple limbs was easier for her to focus on than anything requiring alignment or isolated movement. Static activities like stretching or holding a tough position for an extended period of time were excruciating for her. She hated yoga. Her ideal workout was a free-form dance party in her living room: Beyoncé and beer with a private personal trainer to keep her on task, booty-shaking to the beat.

She was in constant pain of one kind or another. She had excruciating wrist pain from gripping her red correction pen as if she had to physically squeeze the ink out of it while grading papers. The pain in her wrist made its way up her arm into her neck and eventually her jaw. Her doctor gave her a brace, but it didn't help. She had problems sleeping and often ended up on the couch all night with the dogs piled on top of her and reality TV humming in the background. Sleeping on the couch made her neck pain worse which inflamed the jaw and wrist further.

She leapt from one frenetic activity to another, raging from midnight shopping for stickers and pencils at the Walgreen's discount aisle to digging through boxes of papers in her car in search of random articles she was excited to show me. Eventually, her body would break down and leave her sleep walking for days at a time, wrapped in her husband's sweatpants, mismatched socks, heavy sweaters, and blankets, flattened by exhaustion. Thirty minutes passed after we finished our sessions before I could make my escape—ten feet from the base of the staircase to the front door. Her energy rose and fell and rose and fell.

Somehow within this madness Georgia found seemingly limitless stamina to focus on diet and exercise. She went to her diet meetings and stuck to their frozen and boxed food. She worked out with me reliably and maintained the cardio program I gave her to do on her own time. Over the course of those first nine months, she lost sixty pounds. She went from 185 to 125 as her reunion weekend approached.

It worked. Her manic, obsessive pursuit of weight loss was a rollicking success—until the obsession faded; motivation fell away; and the weight returned in force.

Georgia went to the reunion and showed them all how thin she was, but when she got home, the whole routine fell to pieces. She went off of her eating program and started missing appointments with me. She didn't have a cell phone because she was afraid she wouldn't put the phone down while driving (a valid concern), so when she decided not to show up for a session, she simply didn't show. No call, no warning.

Within a few months, she was missing every other appointment. She stayed at work long past our 7 p.m. start time; fixated on her classroom for hours without getting anything organized; and left me parked in her driveway, waiting to see if her headlights might come speeding around the corner. She paid for every missed session but seemed uninterested in either showing up on time or quitting altogether. She lost track of the cardinal rule of wellness and weight loss—consistency—and her body paid the price.

She ran like the energizer bunny all day, drinking diet coke every chance she got and stopping for a burger and large fries on her way home. When she did make it to an appointment, she collapsed into a state of fatigue as soon as she stepped onto the treadmill. Our sessions had always been stop-and-start because of her stories, but eventually the distractions were so intrusive we were lucky to complete two or three exercises in an hour.

Her dedication to the cause was lost. The goal had been reached and passed, and her approach from the beginning was unsustainable; it was far too difficult to maintain. I asked if she would like to quit, but she didn't want to. It would feel like giving up, so we went on like that for months.

When her friends planned another reunion getaway, her obsession began again. She recommitted for a few weeks before deciding that the climb was too steep, especially since the gains from the first time had been so fleeting. She jumped in for one good workout here and there, followed by three days of fast food. She was all over the place, and I never knew which Georgia would appear on any given day.

In spite of her ups and downs, she was a joy to be around. She was funny and enthusiastic, and watching her lose ground after putting in so much effort was extremely difficult. From the outside, it looked like she made incredible progress, but in the process of compartmentalizing and reducing her body, she lost contact with it altogether.

She felt victorious attending the reunion at 125 pounds. The initial motivation to lose weight for the big event was clearly effective. She fought like a woman possessed for that one battle but never took the time to notice what hunger or nourishment felt like, to notice that she actually felt quite full when she piled her plate high with fruits and vegetables. She didn't take the time to notice how her body felt as it moved down past 170 pounds, past 160 and 150.

The goal she set was only barely attainable: 125 pounds was too low for her to comfortably maintain. It required an austere diet, which she had no intention of sustaining over the long haul. She couldn't enjoy any of the food she loved or relax, drinking beers with her husband while he watched football and she read her celebrity rags.

At five foot seven, she could have been very comfortable at 140 or 150 pounds, but she was determined to lose as much as possible. She set a goal, achieved it, and checked it off the list. Once the reunion was over, she threw her hands up in resignation and jumped headlong into a bag of fish and chips. She never noticed on the way back up that 140 might suit her just fine. It was diet food or fast food, success or failure, nothing in between. She blew past 150, headed straight for the 170s.

Her physicality changed as she got bigger, but the weight wasn't even the issue. She couldn't understand where her inspiration went, why weight loss had been so easy and was suddenly so hard. She decided work was bringing her down. She said the commute was too long and the politics at school were too thick for her to stay focused, but none of those things were any different when she was losing weight. She used to make the long drive home after a frustrating day and go for a twenty-minute speed-walk, even on days I wasn't around. But not anymore.

She never paid attention to the fact that those walks helped her sleep better and alleviated her stress and back pain. She never noticed the effects that eating better and moving more had on her quality of life. The changes she made were completely driven by impressing her friends on that one specific weekend with total disregard for her body as a resource.

She never recognized that her body had been dramatically and effectively fine-tuned to facilitate the rest of her life. Instead, it was a finished product to present at the reunion, and when the presentation was complete, she set it aside to gather dust, neglected and bent out of shape.

I doubt that I (or my body) figured into Georgia's thought process, but watching her go through all of this was a roller coaster ride for me too. In addition to being frustrated for her, I had to fight the urge to *keep up* with her. At her lowest weight, I couldn't help feeling like my own client had outdone me. I didn't feel like I could set an example because I was suddenly large in comparison. I thought her progress should have been inspiring, a powerful motivator for me to lose weight right alongside her. We didn't know yet that she would gain it back, but something in the frenzy told me to stay out of the fray.

Her body had nothing to do with mine. I realized that I would much rather be a little heavier than I might wish—but balanced, well fed, and fit—than super-thin for one event and panicked about maintaining an unsustainably low weight. The example I needed to set didn't have anything to do with my weight. More than anything, Georgia needed to witness a measured approach, an appreciation for my body as it was, and a dedication to consistency. I did not try to match her, and as she regained it all, I held steady. Steady or bust.

The truth was that I liked a good meal after a hard workout. I liked to eat dark chocolate every night and had no intention of giving that up. My body reflected my life in full, and that was okay with me. I had a choice between competing with her or staying focused on the balance that was beginning to serve me so well. So I supported her as best I could while staying resolutely on my own course.

I took note each day that I felt better when I ate an orange at 4 o'clock in the afternoon rather than starving myself between lunch and dinner. And I took note of what it felt like to raise my arm up over my head on the pillow at night with a dull ache of soreness in my triceps, having awakened a muscle that hadn't been challenged in a while. They were signs of life, and they became the reward in and of themselves.

When my body is functioning and moving, it makes me feel more awake and engaged. When I do nothing and my joints begin to stiffen, it feels like a loss of freedom. Our bodies are the tools that allow us to live our lives to the best of our abilities, to carry out our dreams and ambitions. When we focus incessantly on measuring, tucking, and sucking them in, we're missing the point. The purpose of fitness is to nurture a body that feels comfortable and capable. If the food you eat and the exercise you engage in point to that end, no matter what your weight might be, you are absolutely moving in the right direction.

Yo-yo dieting happens because the changes we are attempting to put in place are either miserable or too far of a stretch. If you feel yourself recoiling from or wanting to lash out against the changes you are trying to put into place, you're probably taking it a step too far; making too many adjustments at once; or pursuing choices that will never keep you happy in the long run.

Ask yourself if the habit changes you're shooting for are things you can see yourself maintaining throughout the rest of your life. If the answer to that question is "no," pull back and try something else. Both dietary and activity-based changes should feel nurturing and enlivening. If that's the case, they will not be hard to maintain. Even if you get distracted and slip for a while, you won't have any trouble returning to them.

There is some debate about the physiological effects of yo-yo dieting, but there is no question that taking drastic measures to lose weight causes fatigue and irritability, and failing to keep it off elicits frustration and feelings of hopelessness.[1] It has also been shown to increase insulin and estrogen levels and decrease muscle mass, priming the dieter to regain all of the weight and more. In the worst scenarios, yo-yo and extreme dieting can increase the likelihood of developing insulin resistance, diabetes, and heart disease.[2]

The best kind of weight loss is slow and steady. A pound or two a week really is the maximum you should be losing if you want better odds of keeping it off—but think about what a pound a week would actually mean in the long run. A client of mine recently lost ten pounds over the course of six months. She was frustrated with how long it was taking until she realized that if she continued on like that, she would finish out the year twenty pounds lighter than she started. Not too shabby, and her new body weight would feel natural and sustainable.

The difference between taking better care of your body so you can look good in a bathing suit or taking better care so you can be more fulfilled and go on to do bigger things is enormous. It's fine to prioritize weight loss if that will help you be more comfortable, but to make it permanent, you have to lose it by stretching and bolstering your quality of life, not striving for some illusory, impossible measure of perfection.

Georgia restricted every creature comfort until she reached her goal, and then, of course, she let loose and binged. She didn't enjoy the process. None of it had anything to do with finding *pleasure* in her body or in the way she spent her time. She started out with perfectly valid motivation but never checked in along the way to see what a difference the changes made. If she had shifted her attention to the incredible benefits she gained early on—by eating appropriate portion sizes and physically working out some of her psychological turmoil—she might have held on to some of the weight loss. She might have found a more sustainable place to land as her weight dropped—low enough to feel invigorated but high enough to allow for living.

As I watched her struggle, I began guiding her at the end of every session to reach up toward the ceiling, pushing her feet down into the ground and stretching as high as she could, feeling her rib cage lifting up off of her abdomen and diaphragm, making space for her lungs to breathe; before flopping over in a forward bend, releasing her knees, allowing her spine to stretch toward the floor as her arms hung limp off of her shoulders; slowly rolling up, tucking her tail bone and stacking one vertebrae on top of the other until the crown of her head rose up above it all: tall, aligned, centered, and strong.

This simple stretch was my quiet attempt to center her in her body, to make her aware of the muscle and bone that held her up and to add value to the flesh she was so desperately trying to manipulate.

Our bodies make our lives possible. To support them and make them more agile, we have to stay present with them, listening as we experiment with best practices, always in search of food and exercise that will make us feel dynamic and awake. Putting our bodies in a vice and squeezing the life out of them until they shrink to fit will bring nothing but backlash.

Getting healthier is about quality of life. It's about serving our bodies the best we can by weaving an intricate tapestry of pleasure, rest, recovery, and motion.

TOOLBOX

Which food makes you feel bad?
What do you eat on a regular basis that reliably makes you feel crappy? It gives you heartburn or makes you queasy or puts you to sleep at inopportune times. Find one of those, and see what happens if you skip it.

Which food makes you feel good, but you never think to make it?
I cube sweet potatoes with the skin still on, toss in a little olive oil, salt and red pepper, and bake them in the oven at 450 degrees for fifteen or twenty minutes. I do the same with frozen, precut broccoli florets. I love both of those foods but forget half the time how easy and delicious they are. The longer the list I have of quick, easy, healthy things like that, the healthier my body is and the less addicted I feel to processed food. Watermelon. Roasted root vegetables. Corn on the cob. Crock pot stew. Need I say more?

What is one aspect of your fitness or diet plan where you are pushing too hard?
It hurts or you don't like it. Stop.

What is one area of your fitness or diet plan where you could push harder, where you feel genuinely prepared to start doing something specific differently?
Take a leap. Take it to the next level. If you don't feel great when you eat dairy, quit it for a week and see what happens. Quit it for real, fully and completely. Don't half-ass it or make excuses. Cut it all out, and see if you feel better.

Or maybe you enjoy going to the gym but are stuck. Talk to a trainer, or go online to find a routine to step it up a notch.

If you love your daily walks but don't feel challenged anymore, jog every other block; do ten walking lunges every five minutes; or try a different route with more hills.

If you're truly ready, step it up a notch!

8

THE TORTOISE TOTALLY WINS

If you've been on a roll with weight loss or taking better care of yourself but lost your momentum somewhere along the way—or if you were never on a roll in the first place—the whole undertaking can seem disheartening and overwhelming. Knowing when or how to start is tough, and if you've watched a massive amount of effort and progress disappear before your eyes like Georgia did, it can feel almost impossible to begin again. If your odds of keeping it off are so slim, what's the point?

My friend, Lisa, lost a hundred pounds a few years ago, before gaining it all back plus twenty. She weighed 329 pounds when she started, and she weighs 349 now, the heaviest she has ever been. I've talked with her about finding things that give her pleasure and doing more of them, but at this point, at that level of defeat, that approach feels like a microscopic drop in the bucket. It seems insufficient, like it wouldn't get her anywhere at all.

In her own words, Lisa was always the quintessential "fat kid." The other kids on the bus called her "pork chop" in grade school, but she describes her childhood as relatively normal in regards to her body image. She didn't think much about it. She surrounded herself with close friends all the way through high school and college and never felt ostracized. It didn't occur to her until she was in her early twenties that "people would ever think badly of someone because of their body type or weight."

She was never athletic but always loved to swim. She claims that the most she exercised in college was in the middle of a mosh pit, and though she found herself there regularly, slam dancing every once in a while wasn't enough to counteract the gas station food that she ate during the epic road trips she and her friends took to get to far-flung rock shows.

In her family life, her little brother passed away during her senior year in college from acute alcohol poisoning. He was a straight-laced kid who never touched alcohol in high school but went to a friend's twenty-first birthday party one night and tragically drank too much. The loss was devastating.

Lisa worked a series of unfulling jobs after graduation and describes waking up in her apartment two years after his death, "feeling really crappy, like an eighty-year-old person getting out of bed in the morning." She was twenty-three years old, 329 pounds, and approaching blood pressure and cholesterol levels that would have required medical intervention. She was tired of feeling sick and didn't want her parents to lose another kid to something preventable, so she signed up for a four-month weight management class at a local university.

The only vegetables her family had in the house while she was growing up were canned green beans and corn. They had a classic meat and potatoes, fried chicken and burgers kind of a diet. To "get healthy," they busted out iceberg wedges with ranch dressing. When she signed up for the class, she didn't know much about healthy eating beyond what she had heard about popular fad diets, and for the first time in that class she realized that there was a way to lose weight without being hungry.

She began to discover food that could be both healthy *and* filling and began walking and doing water aerobics several times a week. She learned the basics and started down a good path. Over the course of the next few months, she lost twenty pounds by making small changes.

Inspired by her success, a well-meaning friend talked her into signing up for a half marathon. Lisa trained for months and completed the half before she ever even considered doing a 5K or 10K. She describes that half marathon as the most miserable thing she had ever done in her life. The day was hot, the course was hilly, and the run was painful. She was alone on the course in the end, as it took her nearly four and a half hours to complete, and she swore never to do another race again. "I hated life afterward and went back to not exercising," she says. "I didn't have another goal in mind. I just basically thought 'this sucks, and I don't want to do it anymore.'"

At a loss about what to do next, she started auditioning for weight loss reality shows. She passed through several rounds of auditions and interviews and got to the point where casting directors pitched her to the executives. The process took months, and by the end, she was convinced that she would be on the show. This opportunity would be her "savior," and in preparation, she stopped trying to lose weight or take care of herself because she figured that the more weight she had to lose, the more likely she would be to win. When she wasn't cast in the end, she was devastated and directionless.

In search of solace, she began reading weight loss blogs, looking for likeminded people who were also struggling with weight, and decided to start one of her own. Online, accountable to her fellow bloggers, she returned to the simple methods she had learned in class. She weighed 329 pounds in March and set a goal to lose thirty pounds by the end of the year by setting small, behavioral goals, a manageable approach.

She ate a balanced diet and combined it with consistent, regular exercise. She chose lean proteins and complex carbs. She ate more fruits and vegetables, fewer unhealthy fats, and less processed food—but nothing was off limits. If she wanted pizza, she would have two slices along with a salad. She allowed herself to go out with friends and have fun but drank less alcohol than before, which cut calories and had the additional benefit of helping her make better choices with food (both while drinking and the morning after). She was vigilant but not punitive with herself.

By getting back to basics, she began steadily losing weight again. She set her goal in March and hit it by November.

Triumphant at 299 pounds, she was dating a fellow weight loss blogger who convinced her to sign up for another half marathon—which, by the end of the following year, ballooned to *five* half marathons with a sprint triathlon or two thrown in for good measure. The relationship didn't survive, but they did complete the first race they signed up for and remained friends.

Her initial motivation for racing again was to stand by her boyfriend as he struggled with his own weight, and after they broke up, she pressed on to show him what he was missing. The motivation was effective, but, like Georgia, she never stepped back to check in with her body along the way. She got down to 229, but not for long.

Her focus switched entirely to training, and the new eating habits she had worked so hard to develop began to fall apart. Food became secondary. Rather than rewarding her lighter, fitter body with more of the food that transformed it in the first place, she went back to eating whatever she wanted whenever she wanted, including a lot of emotional eating.

By the end of the fifth half marathon, she was gaining weight again, and her body was used up. She was tired and overextended with recurring ankle injuries. She was unhappy at work and single again. The races were not helping her break through the plateau, and in spite of having lost a hundred pounds, she was still profoundly dissatisfied with her body.

At her heaviest, she was under the classic and understandable assumption that her weight was at the root of her problems and that if she lost it, life would be infinitely easier. When she actually did lose it, things were pretty much the same, and she still didn't like what she saw in the mirror. Frustrated, she swore off racing yet again, grew apathetic, and devolved completely into old eating habits.

"There was never a big decision to eat all the things and stop exercising," she said. "It was just a slow progression of turning back to food to feel better. Looking back though, it was probably one of the happiest times in my life. I just wasn't self-aware enough to see what I had accomplished and how much fun I was having." At her lightest, she was swimming, rafting, and hiking on a regular basis; she even went zipling—all activities that are either difficult or impossible now that she has gained the weight back.

She associates her weight loss with racing, which is one reason she has trouble even thinking about taking care of her body again. Those periods of super-human effort shattered the success she was having with moderate exercise and cleaner eating. If she had never signed up for another half marathon—if she had stuck with water aerobics and 5Ks and continued to eat filling, whole food every chance she got—she'd probably be arriving at one hundred pounds down right about now. The weight loss would definitely have taken longer, but a 229-pound body would have been hers for the keeping. She would never have faced the backlash and exhaustion that set her back.

Being back at her highest weight is a difficult place to be. The whole pursuit took years and changed nothing, but she has only been through the cycle of significant weight loss and gain twice, and that process has revealed an identifiable pattern, which gives her an enormous amount of power. Once a pattern is understood, it can be changed.

She thinks the half marathons brought about the weight loss, but, in reality, they subverted it. Each time she embarks on a moderate approach, she loses some weight, starts feeling better, and gets overly ambitious. She leaps too far too fast, exhausts herself, and slides back into the oldest, deepest trench she knows: food as comfort.

She has every tool she needs. She knows how food impacts her and which choices are healthiest. She has the ambition and ability to take better care of herself, and in hindsight, it's clear why she wasn't able to stick with it. She was over-training and under-nourishing. She was ignoring her body's pleas for mercy and missing critical opportunities to revel in her success. Of course, it's difficult to revel in a body that still doesn't feel perfect, but it's crucial to notice and appreciate small breakthroughs, signs of strength and agility, not just the progress reflected on the scale.

She has the skills and information to shape a body that works better for her. The only things missing in the past were patience and consistency. If she can cultivate those, she can do it again—for good this time. There is no reason Lisa can't reach and maintain a more comfortable weight. Maybe she'll end up comfortable at 250 pounds or 280. Everyone's body is different, and there is no *one* ideal weight. Only she will know when she crosses over from feeling liberated to feeling deprived. When that happens, if she can rest for a bit where she is, within a few months she might find that she's prepared to lose a little more, to push through from that new plateau with solid ground underfoot. But if she tries to press on before she is ready, she's almost guaranteed to boomerang right back to where she started.

No matter how much she loses, she won't ever achieve the picture of perfection she holds in her head. None of us ever do, no matter how thin we get. Bodies are imperfect by nature. They're supposed to be that way. They are always works in progress, and their beauty lies in their functionality, not their size. For Lisa, the only finish line worth pursuing is a body limber and light enough to support the life and activities she holds dear.

People who set out on a workout or diet plan with the most intense determination are often the ones who crash and burn. They pick up a heavy backpack full of frustration and set out to climb the tallest mountain around, determined to reach the top by sundown, when it's actually a life-long climb. They don't see results fast enough. Legs start to ache, stomachs start to growl, and they give up in a spectacular display of self-sabotage, sitting down to a pepperoni pizza in a dimly lit room with the flashing blue light of the TV to distract them from the letdown. They don't realize that slow and steady really does win the race. Setting attainable goals that can be maintained for the long haul will set them on a much more successful path.

If you're striving for a body you can maintain, rapid weight loss is your worst enemy—unfortunate but true. The best and only reliable way to get there is to push as far as you can comfortably go, change however many habits you comfortably can, pause to celebrate and regroup, and then push a little further. It's the tortoise and the hare—and the tortoise totally wins.

The key is incremental forward motion. Overreaching is a recipe for disaster, but so is the other trap people so frequently fall into, the opposite of overreaching: stagnation. Doing too much can break your body and spirit, *but so can doing too little*. Our minds and bodies need stimulation to grow. We are in a constant state of flux. We continually turn over new cells in our skin and muscles. If we challenge them properly—just enough, but not too much—we can fortify those new tissues to support better overall health and a more vibrant appearance.

There is energy in motion in your body whether you know it or not. You grow hair and nails; your heart beats; your lungs breathe; and you get a little bit older every day. You are physically always in the process of evolving. There's no such thing as living static. As you move and grow, if you can find a narrow path between stagnation and overexertion that works for you, you can set yourself perpetually in motion toward a stronger body rather than a stiffer, more sedentary one.

It's a delicate balance, and it changes over time. Running might feel good for a while, until it doesn't. Softball might take over, until soccer, dancing, roller derby, or tai chi begin to look more interesting. It's a forever-changing process, but figuring out your plan as you go can be satisfying, curious, and engaging even. Your focus on your body becomes centered on what makes you feel *better* rather than what might, maybe, someday make you *skinnier*.

In that mindset, you're never asking the question, "Will this food make me fat?" You're asking, "Does this food make my body feel good?" Your mind will continue on with its tricks, telling you that your old standbys are what you want, but as you clue into your body, you'll begin receiving other messages. Listen to the cues as best you can; try different things and make adjustments as you go.

"Failure" will happen. You'll push too far or pursue something you don't end up enjoying in the slightest. It will hurt or bore you to tears, and you'll want to forget the whole thing. Or you might make good strides by taking walks every morning and eating healthier snacks each day, but your weight and sense of wellness will stall.

The weird and wonderful path to wellness is an experiment, and you *will* feel as if you have fallen on your face several times along the way. Your big plan, the one that you were absolutely sure would work, will fall apart. When your guard is down—either because you're on a roll or in the trenches—Lothario will bring you a glass of wine and a pile of brownies. He will envelop you in sweet surrender. "Just for tonight," he'll say.

If you understand that a fleeting binge or a few weeks of lethargy are temporary, if you're willing to let them go, you'll snap out of it, no harm done and get back on track. But if you take it as a personal failure or crushing defeat, you can slip away for days or months at a time and wake up aghast as the scale skyrockets beyond where it began. *Do not deny yourself the right to stumble.* If you do, momentary lapses can gain momentum and grow to be catastrophic.

No matter how far gone you might be, wrap your arms around the process of figuring out what works, and allow it to change over time. There will always be a damn fine excuse not to bother. There will always be an injury, a broken heart, or a demanding job, but if you show up reliably and *do something* that contributes to your well-being— whether depressed or full of energy—you *will* continue getting closer to where you want to be.

Come back to basics; they will extricate you every time. The end-game is freedom, not perfection. A visit with destructive, old habits is a useful reminder and nothing more. To give it any more power than that is a mistake. Recognize what's happening, forgive the backslide, and sidestep it. Keep moving: no guilt, no extreme diets, no punishing work-outs—just back to daily therapy for your body, shaping muscles and ligaments, strong and loose, strong and loose.

The little voice every morning, telling you that preparing a healthy breakfast is too much of a hassle or you can walk tomorrow when you're not so busy, will keep repeating itself. It knows the drill, and it's going to take you to exactly the same place it took you yesterday and the day before that. Go ahead and listen to it—for a day, or a week, or two, until you're ready to lean again on the infrastructure that holds you up.

An arrow has to be pulled back before it can fly. It needs adequate tension to propel itself forward. That tension might be disconcerting, but it can also be extremely helpful. Pay attention to the heaviness as it comes on again. Feel it pulling at you, and recognize it as the uncomfortable but necessary force needed to propel you forward. Take note of it, and turn back to the reliable behavior that you know will pull you toward better and away from worse.

When Lisa hit a hundred pounds down, she felt infinitely better, but the reflection in the mirror and the feel of her new body were nowhere near what she had imagined. She went back into combat with her body instead of elevating it, and with the old condemnation came a familiar and compulsory thirst for the simple satisfaction of a food-induced serotonin rush. In the thick of the fight, she couldn't remember how to stop the freefall. With each additional pound, her condemnation and thirst grew, and she abandoned herself as a lost cause.

But she wasn't a lost cause and still isn't. She just got distracted. She could sense in her heart that what she had accomplished was remarkable, maybe even transcendental, but she couldn't feel any of the jubilation that she expected. Instead, she found a sense of emptiness. Her job and relationship status were the same. The desire to eat still nagged at her. Clothes still fit all wrong, and she was still fifty pounds away from a "normal" BMI. On top of all that, she was exhausted. She pushed too hard for too long and didn't allow herself time for healing.

"Looking back now," she says with water welling in her eyes, "I looked so good, and I felt amazing. I was so healthy, but it wasn't enough. My brain didn't connect with why I was doing this. I know now that there really is no endpoint. It's ongoing. It's about living."

She had weight goals and visions of what her life would be like when she reached them. She relied on the half marathons to keep her on pace and had a master plan for a mythical body. She ended up lighter and leaner, but that wasn't good enough. She didn't feel "right" yet. Desperation led to more intense training which led to exhaustion, and disappointment led back to food.

The freedom to hike and go rafting with friends didn't mean enough at the time to sustain her, but that freedom definitely would now. She can see the process and her challenges clearly and has every resource available to get back there if she takes her time. The arrow has been pulled back to a breaking point, but she knows now, perfectly well, how to let it soar.

Too much exercise and an all-or-nothing approach will sabotage her efforts every time, but if she proceeds with caution, slow and steady, tortoise-style, she will creep along, and every day will be freer than the one before. She'll find a weight that works, a zone of comfort and health, and she'll stay there.

TOOLBOX

What went wrong?

With the benefit of hindsight, now is a good time to figure out what not-so-helpful patterns you have perpetuated over the years. Bust out the journal, and go back through your life, beginning with childhood, looking with broad strokes at the phases you have been through with your body. This isn't about deep analysis. You should be able to scroll through your entire life up to the present on a page or two.

What was your relationship with exercise and food as a kid, an adolescent, and through early adulthood? When did you go into battle against your body? Was that battle related to anything in particular and what tactics did you use? Did they work? If so, did the results last? As years passed, what other methods did you try? When did each battle fall apart, and what happened next? How long did you give up before trying again, and how did those attempts go? What else was happening when you started getting somewhere, and what else was happening when your plan began falling apart?

The idea here is to get a clear picture of your patterns in general terms so you can stop the destructive ones from taking over again when they arise by turning back to the archive of healthy habits you're generating. If clarity on this doesn't come easily, don't stress about it. Come back to it later. Over time it will get clearer.

Set new parameters, other than weight loss, to judge your progress by.

What positive results do you see and feel in your body from healthy changes you are making right now? Even if your weight seems perpetually stuck, take note of the physical and psychological benefits you are getting from treating your body right. This stuff matters, and the list can include anything.

Is it easier to walk up stairs or get up off the floor? Feeling strong? Does your back hurt less? Are you less sleepy mid-afternoon? Have cravings subsided during a specific time of day? Have you nurtured a friendship by going out for a walk with someone? Are you less likely to snap at your coworkers or kids? Do you feel more confident? Are you sleeping better? Is your skin clearer? Are you getting up the guts to ask for a raise at work or to propose a new project?

If you are writing your list of three glimpses of blue sky each day, add a few of these improvements to the list. Give your body some love. Focus on the progress you've made. Health is about *so much more* than weight loss. If you waste all of your time focusing on weight, you'll miss the opportunity to notice how much better you feel in all kinds of ways.

Get your head in the right place around "special occasions."

A special occasion is something that happens once a year or once a decade: your birthday, an anniversary, a graduation, or a promotion. That's about it. Those are the only occasions worth blowing it out for—and, even then, the whole idea of "blowing it out" is questionable.

First of all, there is no reason—ever—to eat so much that you feel sick or lethargic, *especially* not on a special occasion. Why would you want to do that to yourself when you need energy for celebrating and want to feel at your best?

Second, if you include holidays, office parties, travel, conferences, concerts, cookouts, happy hours, and every wedding, birthday, bachelorette party, bridal shower, baby shower, bitch-fest, and dance party you attend, you can rest assured that you will almost never get through a week without being obligated to attend some sort of blow-out worthy occasion. So where does that leave you? Stuffed and unhappy.

It is absolutely possible to be social; show up for every event; thoroughly enjoy yourself; and *also* eat and drink for energy and lightness. Just because you're at a party doesn't mean you have to stuff your face. Have a taste of anything you want, and leave it at that. Stopping with a few bites or turning down that last cocktail is so much easier when normal, hum-drum days are not full of restrictions. If regular days are enjoyable too and parties aren't associated with cheating, you won't feel driven to eat as much as possible while you're in "cheat mode." There won't be any such thing as cheat mode. Going to a party and having fun don't have to be synonymous with eating too much.

9

DO SOMETHING

So what happens when you've had enough? You're sick of feeling stuck, but the adjustments you've made don't seem to be leading anywhere. What can you change in your diet and fitness routine that will make a lasting difference without freaking you out?

Before you make any grand goals, any big purchases of equipment, any promises to yourself or your family, stop and ask yourself if you can be happy with your body the way it is.

Some of us who tend to worry about weight and body image might forget that many people live their whole lives happily, healthfully plump—and a lot of them are more fit than you might imagine. They exercise and eat healthy home-cooked meals. They have stellar careers and fulfilling relationships. They feel good overall and have made their peace with the extra weight. Bottom line, they enjoy life on their own terms. They eat and drink freely, and if a little extra weight is the price they have to pay to maintain that lifestyle, it's a trade they're willing to make.

I don't know about you, but I prefer the company of people who are at peace with themselves over those who are not, no matter their size. I would so much rather hang with somebody who is big and fun than with someone thin and dismal.

On any given day, in any given moment, you have a choice between engaging in the same habits you always have, that perpetuate the same body, or making changes that will bring about a different one. Both options are valid. In addition to everything you've already tried, this chapter will provide you with some specific steps to take, but here's the thing: there is *no reason* to torture yourself with weight goals if you're not ready to push past your comfort zone to pursue them or if they don't matter to you all that much to begin with.

If you decide to carry on as you are, do so joyfully with an open heart. Make that choice, and be that person without apology. Live in your body in the healthiest way you can, free of self-recrimination. Focus your wellness goals on strength, flexibility, and energy, not pounds lost. Walk as much as you can. Lift light weights, do squats or modified push-ups (knees on the ground) a few times a week to increase bone density and muscle strength, and stretch on a regular basis to maintain flexibility. Just a few easy adjustments can be enough to help you feel better and prevent disease and injury, at least to some degree.

If, on the other hand, you want to feel lighter, if it has become more important for you to feel *different* than to be comfortable, different choices will have to be made several times a day, every day. If that's the case, understand that differentness feels odd. Making a change in diet or exercise can throw you off in ways that seem unrelated. It can affect your sleep or work patterns, attitudes and relationships in ways you never anticipated.

Making haphazard changes across the board is a recipe for failure. Continue to pinpoint which changes you can realistically maintain and which, in all honesty, you're not ready to address. The process will be hit or miss—requiring you to jump, shift, and change tactics until you figure out what gets results.

When I started working through this process myself, I hiked up a hill every day. That was the extent of what I knew I could successfully accomplish, and that was all. I knew I could do it (and maintain my commitment to it) because it felt good. Moving and breathing were rewarding in and of themselves, weight loss aside. Sometimes the hikes were ten minutes, and sometimes they were two hours. Most of the time it was somewhere in between, but I did it almost every day. I still ate too much late at night. Worrying over this or that, I needed that tried and true habit to soothe my nerves. I needed the comfort and resigned myself to how it would affect my weight—but hiking was something productive I could do, something new. I didn't know how I'd ever end up in a place that felt easy without empty late-night snacks, but I had my eye on the prize. That almost unimaginable freedom was my grand objective, and the hikes kept me moving in the right direction.

The end goal was to *make peace* with my body, regardless of how long it took, so I put one foot in front of the other up the hill—one solid habit to reinforce my well-being—and over the years, I supplemented that habit with more. Nutrition classes were taken; books were read; healthy snacks were added; candy bars were subtracted; the gym membership got used; and my mind took a rest from the incessant debate over what I should or should not eat. One habit grew to four, five, and six—until my body and mind were unrecognizable from where they started.

So, where should you begin, and how far can you push? What is realistic? The answer shouldn't have anything to do with how much weight you hope to lose in the next year. Instead, just do everything you can—on every front you can—to feel better and get stronger. Figure out which new behavior you can build into your life right now that will stick and blossom into others.

This chapter will provide you with two sets of tips, physical and psychological reinforcements, tactics to try and methods to lean on as you go. (Side note: if you've read enough books with enough tips for a lifetime and are sick of this crap, skip straight to chapter 10.)

You can approach these changes cold turkey or in slow motion. For the greatest effect, I recommend a combination of the two. Some scabs are better ripped off and left to bleed while others need to be nurtured and bandaged until they are ready to fall off on their own. The trick is knowing which is which. Purposefully decide which habits you don't need anymore, and which you do. When you get ready, rip the scabs off of the ones you don't need. Walk away from them, and decisively hang on to those you do still need. They will bring you relief as the others fall away, leaving you groundless and making room for your body to change.

You're building your protective pod. The steely infrastructure at the center is a collection of a few accessible habits that will clear your head and lift your mood without fail every time you turn to them. This chapter is devoted to those core habits. Try each suggestion to see which comes naturally, and continue to pad the exterior of your pod with softness, compassion for hits and misses; cushy old comforts and dear friends to keep you sane.

Georgia could make a commitment to bring snacks to eat in the car on the way home from work and swear off the takeout that helped her pack the weight back on. And she could also set a date with her husband to go out for fish and chips on the last Sunday of every month, a throwback to her childhood that she could look forward to. Change one thing, and keep another.

There are probably several things in your life that you are ready to leave behind. At this point, you're just doing them by rote and wouldn't be all that brokenhearted to never do them again. Whatever those habits are, be done with them, and don't look back. Stop ordering egg rolls with your stir-fry. Stop watching the reality show you *don't* like just because the one you *do* like isn't airing this month. Stop going home right after work on Monday nights and go directly to the gym instead. Replace the potato chips in your lunch bag with unsalted cashews. Make a few mini-changes and live with them for a minute before digging into more difficult territory.

It's like cleaning out your closet. Get rid of the junk you know you don't need first, before turning your focus to items that require a little more consideration, that may or may not fit or hold a bit of sentimental value. Once you've cleared out the clutter, you can see more easily which remaining habits you would like to change and how to go about it.

The initial shake-up will feel like progress and give you momentum to keep pushing further. Beyond that, aim small; be consistent; and move slowly but steadily forward with one or more of the following suggestions.

Little things add up. If you eat two hundred fewer calories and walk one thousand more steps per day for an extended period of time, you *will* lose weight. Your energy balance will be different, and your body will change. Once that first new behavior is second nature, if you're inspired, one-up yourself. Add something else, maybe something a little more challenging. When you start to get high from feeling different in your skin, you'll crave more of it. It's not about running marathons. It's about regularly pushing one step beyond where you already are.

The following is a list of ten simple tips that also happen to be game-changers. You've probably heard all of them before. You might have dismissed them among the heap of diet tips and schemes that come across your radar every day, but they do make a difference if you stick with them. And if you approach them as ways to free yourself from destructive, old habits rather than limitations you're required to abide by, pursuing them might even feel good. They seem simple, but they have reliably helped me and my clients lose weight or, at least, feel much better. They will help you uproot your routine. Try them on for size, and see if any might be long-term solutions that can change your life and body for the better.

1. Never eat in front of the television or computer. Just don't. It will distract you from how much food you are putting in your mouth and from whether or not you're full. It will allow you to ingest enormous amounts of calories unchecked and unconsciously.

2. Always eat breakfast and watch the sugar. Sugar will mess you up first thing in the morning. It will spike your blood sugar and trigger cravings throughout the day. If you want something sweet, do it with fresh, whole fruit and some kind of protein. Breakfast should always include fiber and protein. Fiber will aid digestion and slow down your insulin response. Protein keeps you feeling full longer. Have peanut butter or almond butter on whole grain toast or an apple. Have unsalted nuts with a few dried cranberries, low-fat cottage cheese with fruit, egg whites with spinach, onions, and tomatoes, or low-sugar/high-fiber cereal with fresh berries and skim, soy, or almond milk. Don't assume that healthy food has to taste like cardboard. Keep looking until you find options you like, and eat in the morning even if you aren't hungry. Eating breakfast wakes up your brain, gets your metabolism and digestive system going at the beginning of the day, and reduces the likelihood that you will make destructive choices later.

Nutritionists used to believe that losing weight was a matter of calories in versus calories out, but new studies have shown that we have something called "clock genes" that cause us to burn more calories and more fat, more efficiently, earlier in the day.[1] Front load the calories in your day as much as you can, and *stop eating at least two or three hours before bed.* This kind of switch can have an enormous impact on your weight. Even if you can't stand eating much in the morning, make lunch your big meal of the day instead of dinner.

3. Snack. Eat enough to take the edge off of your hunger, especially in the middle of the afternoon. This boosts your metabolism and keeps you satisfied so you don't gorge yourself at dinner and afterward. It also keeps your energy and focus consistent throughout the day. Think fresh food over prepackaged whenever possible. Small amounts: one to two hundred calories. An apple, banana, Greek yogurt, carrots and hummus, celery and peanut butter, unsalted nuts—any of those work. If you have to eat an "energy bar," make sure it has low-sugar content and a decent amount of protein and fiber, but as much as you can, try to eat whole food for your snacks rather than processed, packaged food.

4. Pack your lunch as often as possible, and eat dinner at home. Going out to restaurants packs on fat, sodium, sugar, and calories when you don't even realize it. Eating in saves money too, though, admittedly, cooking after work can be a pain. Try a crock pot or make casseroles in advance that can be eaten for several days. Make a large portion of steamed or sautéed vegetables on Sundays that can be packed for lunch or incorporated into meals throughout the week. Do a little preplanning over the weekend to make weekdays as easy as possible. And if you do end up eating out a lot, think about how you can order lighter. Change the sauce/dressing; eat leaner meats; lose the cheese or sour cream; skip the bread or appetizers; or split your main course with a friend.

5. Reduce portion sizes. You do *not* need to clean your plate. This is, by far, the most effective way to cut back on calories without feeling deprived. You can still have the food you love, just have a little less. Restaurant or take-out meals can stretch to two meals. Keep the leftovers for another night or lunch the next day, or just leave a little more on your plate than usual and walk away. When eating at home, use smaller plates. Have your pasta, but throw a bunch of extra veggies in the sauce and eat three-quarters of what you normally would. Try whole wheat or quinoa pasta; you'll get full faster, and your blood sugar won't spike as high. Same goes for desserts; don't deprive yourself, but watch the portions.

Beware of foods you know you can't stop eating. If you know that a particular food or restaurant causes you to lose control, you may have to cut it out completely, at least for a little while. I don't like to take anything off the table, but there are some things that we are simply powerless to stop eating when they are in front of us. Do not put yourself up against a temptation you know you can't resist. Avoiding it preemptively might be your best option until your desires and taste buds have time to change.

6. Watch out for liquid calories like soda, beer, smoothies, and coffee with cream and sugar. Most people can easily cut out several hundred calories per day in liquids. Drink club soda with a splash of juice instead of soft drinks, or put low-fat milk in your coffee instead of cream. Small sacrifices. Eventually, you might come to like the new choice even better. I promise that actually does happen! And drink water, water, and more water. People often mistake thirst for hunger. Try drinking water before you reach for a snack, and see if you're still hungry in ten minutes. Water is also good for the function of every organ in your body including your skin, which will be softer and clearer if you are well hydrated.

A note about diet soda. I have had something verging on addiction to diet soda since I was about fifteen years old, so if you drink it, you will get no judgment from me. But in recent years, the onslaught of research about its deleterious effects finally convinced me to give it up (except once or twice a year when I get wacky like that). Sweet and bubbly as it might be, studies have shown that diet soda consumption is correlated with a decrease in vital gut bacteria that helps us process sugar, increased belly fat, increased risk of heart disease, and decreased bone density (osteoporosis).[2] Additionally, because artificial sweeteners are many hundreds of times sweeter than sugar, diet soda seems to decrease our sensitivity to real sugar, making us desire much more than normal to get even a low level of satisfaction from it. As with much of nutritional science, nothing is definitive; everything is continually being evaluated. There are lots of mitigating factors in all of these studies, but overall it appears that soda (diet or otherwise) is harmful to your health (and your figure). It just isn't worth it. Go for seltzer with a splash of juice instead; still sweet, still sparkly.

7. Eat as many whole foods as you can, especially fruits and vegetables. Reduce the amount of processed, packaged food you are taking in by adding good stuff to crowd out the bad. Whole grains, fresh fruits, raw, steamed, and sautéed veggies (sauté in olive oil with herbs and spices), unsalted nuts (salt can trigger cravings), whole fresh cheeses, tofu (try "baked" if you don't like the consistency), lean meats and poultry (organic if you can afford it), and fish (download a pocket guide of good fish choices from the Monterey Bay Aquarium or get their iPhone/Android app).[3] The fresher the food the better. You are not likely to overdo it on apples and oranges any time soon.

Even switching from Doritos to BBQ flavor whole grain rice chips or quinoa chips can add fiber and begin shifting your palate. I have had a lot of success counseling clients to trade their favorite snack foods for the health food store versions. They like them enough to feel satisfied, but not so much that they lose control and eat the whole package all at once.

8. Look for *high fructose corn syrup* and *partially hydrogenated oil* and avoid them like the plague. They are in bread, crackers, salad dressings, and frozen foods. Basically, they are in the majority of packaged foods, but not all of them. It is possible to find packaged food without these two ingredients. You just have to look. Thankfully, some major food producers are finally cutting these ingredients out.

High fructose corn syrup has been shown to cause more weight gain than regular sugar, as well as a higher percentage of belly fat and heart damaging triglycerides.[4] Partially hydrogenated oil raises bad cholesterol levels (LDL) and lowers good cholesterol (HDL), which increases your overall risk of heart disease.[5] There's just no reason to put any of that into your body. See the endnotes from Princeton researchers and the Mayo Clinic to read more about how and why these two additives are destructive to your health.

9. Set specific times during the week to exercise and do not let yourself off the hook. Set an alarm on your phone to remind you the night before to get ready. Choose something you can enjoy. Take a ten-minute walk if that's where you need to start. Make an appointment with a trainer if you need to be accountable to someone or need guidance on correct form and how to use machines. Meet a friend at the gym or have her over to your house every Wednesday at 5:30 p.m. for aerobics on-demand in the living room. When your friends, family, and coworkers ask you to make plans during those times, say no. Those days and times of the week have to be non-negotiable. You are going to the gym or the park or the stairs, whatever. You go. Period.

Make those little bits of exercise as important as showing up for work. Pick someone to whom you can send a text or email to confirm you've done it. They don't even need to respond. They only need to receive. Choose a combination of activities and spread them out over the course of the week. Mix it up. Take a yoga or spinning class, jog a block and walk a block and do it again, run for speed on a treadmill for thirty-second intervals, get on the elliptical, lift some weights, play racquetball, go hiking, go biking, go swimming, find a tennis court, walk around the mall, play ping-pong. Don't do exactly the same thing over and over again for months on end. You will get bored and your body will stop adapting.

10. Get some sleep. Going to bed an hour earlier than usual every night can transform your body. Sleep reduces cortisol levels, the stress hormone that makes you think you're hungry when you're not, causes blood sugar levels to spike, and increases body fat storage.[6] Also, when you're exhausted, making good decisions is even harder than usual. You think you need quick energy from carbs when in fact all you need is a little more sleep. Plus, one hour less of wakeful time at night affords less opportunity for snacking after dinner.

Those are my practical, sensible, reasonable tips that you've probably heard a million times. You read them and think, "Yes! I can do that!"—and then nothing happens. Implementing them, actually picking three or four to circle on the page and build into your life, is another story, especially if you have "failed" repeatedly in the past.

If you have always eaten in front of the television, doing mealtime differently won't be easy. The silence can be deafening, a venture into the unknown. And eating three-quarters of your normal portion size isn't easy either. Great in theory, but doing it, regularly, for weeks and months until it becomes habitual is another thing.

So how do you actually execute those changes and make them stick? The next set of ten tips is a concise review of the techniques you have been developing throughout the book. They will help you decide if and when you're ready to actually *do* something and give you techniques to hang on to when your motivation drifts beyond your grasp.

1. Revisit old habits. When you forget why you're making all of these difficult changes to begin with, remind yourself by going back to revisit the bad habit in a controlled, conscious way. Give yourself permission for twenty-four hours to wallow in them fully *and unapologetically* until you're ready to be done with them. Feel the satisfaction and dull nausea as you get ready for bed at night after eating a tub of Ben & Jerry's and half a bag of chips, and get frustrated the next morning as you squeeze into clothes that are uncomfortably tight. Make a vow to go on a raw food diet for the day, skip lunch, and then get too much of your favorite takeout on the way home. Wash it down with a bag of cookies. Purposefully familiarize yourself all over again with how those choices make you feel. Do it without putting a guilt trip on yourself, and get back on track before too much damage is done.

2. Get pissed off. Get pissed at the restaurants that flash commercials in your face every day making you believe that a meat lover's pizza will make you feel social and lively! Get pissed at the food manufacturers who spend millions on research to figure out how to make their food cheap and addictive. And get pissed at the billboards, magazines, TV shows, and movies that equate being freakishly thin with being happy and powerful.I don't know about you, but I resent the implication that I need to be ultra thin to be beautiful and successful. I battled with my body every day for years so I could fit my average-build hips into a size two miniskirt, but of course, I never did and never will. The difference now is that I don't want to anymore. I don't regret a lot of things in life, but I do regret every bit of energy I have wasted beating myself up for not being "skinny" enough, and I mourn the years lost worrying about my weight rather than enjoying being young and healthy. I resent the idea that my self-worth should be attached to how thick or thin I am, and I think you should resent it too. Let acceptance of your body be an act of defiance. Take control back, and determine your own criteria for happiness and well-being.

3. If you must set a weight goal, make it a *range* that you are comfortable with. Set a *realistic* goal, usually a range of five to fifteen pounds is a good idea. Think long and hard about where this range should sit. It should be light enough that you can feel vibrant, but high enough that you can maintain it without avoiding chocolate for the rest of your life or trying to become athlete of the year. Find a range that fits you, not what your mother thinks you should weigh or even necessarily what *you* always thought you should weigh. Look at it with fresh eyes.

At the bottom of the range, you should feel like you have won, you are in a shining moment. At the top of the range, you should be happy and feel good in your clothes, healthy and alive. Once you have maintained this range for a few months and it begins to feel natural, you can reevaluate how you feel to see if going lower would bring any real benefit. Know that the range will change over time, and it may not feel like you thought it would when you get there. Be flexible until you find a good landing place, and always, always, always couple any weight loss goals with strength-based ones.

If my very first client, Diane, could have set a goal to bench press thirty pounds rather than to *lose* thirty pounds, when she did it, she would have felt a sense of accomplishment. The next goal could have been to squat thirty pounds. Goals should be proactive, not punitive. The self-degradation she was battling was so powerful that the thought of losing even five pounds seemed insurmountable. If she had focused on strength instead, she would have realized that she had the capacity to succeed and the power to have an impact on her body.

4. Make sure you dig your new habit. Somehow, someway you better like it. If you're replacing your morning muffin with something healthier, it better be something you enjoy, or you will be back to the muffin before noon. Don't try to replace steak cordon bleu and scalloped potatoes with boiled chicken and steamed cauliflower. If you do, you're begging to fail. Pick foods and activities that you like (at least a little bit). If you can find something to love, you're set. And know this: Exercise is not a horrible, annoying thing you have to do to be thin. *It is the most impactful thing you can do to set yourself free.*

5. Be *stubborn*. When you catch yourself saying, "I'm too tired," "I'm too busy," "The kids are too demanding," "Work is too much," "I've been on this stupid treadmill for eight minutes, and there's no way in hell I'm going to make it to fifteen," *get stubborn with yourself.* Refuse to listen. Put your head down and plow through for two more minutes, then two more after that. Recognize that this kind of defeatist self-talk is *not real*. Your mind is playing tricks on you, repeating the thought patterns that have kept you in your current condition for years.

Ignore yourself. If you've made it eight minutes, you can make it seven more. Keep taking steps until you reach your goal for the day. Be as stubborn with yourself now as you were with your parents when you were sixteen. This is your life, and this is what you want. It's an activity you chose because you liked it, so *refuse* to listen to the bullshit in your head telling you that you can't do it—and then go do it, because then it will be done, and you'll be the champion in gym shorts, jiggly and sweaty and all.

6. Go cheeseball. When you're done being pissed off and you have moved on to implementing changes, spend time dreaming about what life would be like if you found yourself in a younger version of your ideal old lady body, sooner rather than later. Take two minutes of your drive time, your waiting-in-line time, or your shower time to put energy and focus on how it would feel to be in a body that works for you, not just what it would look like, but how it would *feel* in your heart and in your skin. Think about it before bed or when you wake up in the morning. And put steady focus on what you want to accomplish *outside* of fitness and weight loss. Spend a little time and energy on the liberation you'd like to see, instead of on doubts and anxiety. Go all new agey. And then go out, and get on with it.

7. Find motivation that works. Why exactly do you want to change your body? Really and truly? As I've said, it doesn't have to be pretty. Revenge is one of my favorites. When I was dating Antonio, I took every bit of anger and resentment I had and used it for motivation to prove to him (and myself) how fit I could get. If you have some spare anger lying around, channel it.

If not, pick a child, a parent, or somebody you love who you want to be *better* for, and then put on your sneakers and put one foot in front of the other—but do a real gut check on it. The motivation you choose should be something you're actively *thirsting* for. Find what matters to you in the deepest place in your heart, not what is supposed to matter but what really truly matters, and put some physical reminder of it on your desktop, your mirror, or phone. *Plant a very specific image of someone or something in your mind and lean on it* when you can't summon the energy to get up and out. Use it. Sear it into your brain. Find the thing that you want to be fit and healthy for—your kids, your career, your longevity, your peace of mind, your God, pissing off your ex-boyfriend. Whatever the motivation, go back to that one, specific thing and pull it up to the front of mind when you are feeling weak and distracted. Find what matters, and leverage it.

8. Give back. Do as many nice things for other people as you can. Volunteering and donating money to good causes are wonderful things to do, but it's also important to be kind and compassionate to people you encounter in the world at large, even on a bad day, maybe even more so on a bad day. Hold the door open for an invisible, middle-aged man at the drug store who has probably never had a door held open for him in his life. Smile at the woman who sells you your newspaper in the morning. Buy a purse from a fair trade website that will send the money back to the artisan in a developing nation, instead of buying one from a department store. If you're stressed out and stuck, shake things up by being as kind and helpful as you can. Being kinder feels better. It gets you out of your own head and dependably brings interesting new people into your life who can help you see things from a fresh perspective.

Example: I almost caused a terrible car accident by pulling into oncoming traffic a couple of months ago. I was heartbroken and distracted because my grandfather was in the hospital and slipping quickly. The man driving the other car screeched to a halt, inches from my passenger door. He locked eyes with me and waved me on, shaking his head generously and mouthing, "Don't worry. It's okay." I want to be like that guy as often as possible, to give people the benefit of the doubt. He gave it to me, and there's no reason why I can't give it to somebody else. You never know whose Papa might be in the hospital.

9. If you need a fudge brownie, go get a fudge brownie. I mean if you *need* fudge, go get it. Don't do it on every little whim and don't buy a whole pan, but if you are thinking about it and obsessing about it, go get it from someplace special in a reasonable portion size; bring it back home; and eat it without reservation. Enjoy it, guilt-free.

10. Don't think too much. Put your attention on the actions of your body. Forget about uncovering how and why all of your habits or heartbreak came to pass. That's a whole lot of mayhem that could (and probably will) take a lifetime to sort out. I don't know about you, but a lifetime is too long for me to wait to start doing something about feeling better. Don't push the mess down or pretend it's not there. Let it be, but take its power away. Put focus on your body, and let your feet do the walking. Don't anticipate the gym and how hard it's going to be. Just get there and start moving, even if you imagine you'll only have the energy to walk a slow half of a mile. Get there, and do it.

Bring your attention back to the body. If you find yourself caught in patterns of snacking uncontrollably and coming to your senses with an empty box of cookies on your lap and nachos crumbled all over your shirt, look at your hands. Catch the moment when your hands are reaching for the snack or picking up the phone to call for delivery. Catch it. Pause. Look at your hands. Take a deep breath, and make a conscious decision about whether or not to proceed. Go ahead and fulfill the craving, but at the very least, stop long enough to be aware of what you are doing. Over time, making a different choice will get easier.

Use your eyes to see your hands. Use your feet to take you through the door of the gym. Don't think too much. The body is concrete, and if you give it decent instructions, it will not let you down.

When I decided to kick Antonio's ass with my fabulousness, I set my mind on getting to the gym. I found workout plans online and followed them to the letter. I proceeded by rote. Gym. Period. No thinking; no room for debate.

Six a.m. Alarm clock goes off like a knife through the skull. Fling an arm over to reach for the off button. Knock over water glass. Scare the cat. Take a deep breath in through the nose. Repeat. Sit upright, still breathing. Reach for workout clothes placed by the bed the night before and get changed under the covers. Turn on the light, get out of bed, and put on sneakers. Stumble to the kitchen and drink chocolate soy milk out of the carton. Feel sugar hitting the brain. Feed cat while brewing tea. Grab travel mug, prepacked duffel bag with change of clothes and shower supplies, prepacked apple, breakfast bar, and lunch. Put on sunglasses even if the sun is only partially up. Get into the car and drive to the gym. Every day, without fail, I felt more alive by the time I sat down at my desk at 9 a.m.

Whatever habit you choose, implement it. Don't consider your options. Just get there. Drag your groggy, angry, sleepy self to the track; around the block; or to the produce section. Show up. It will be the most remarkable, mundane thing you have ever done, and it will begin to change everything.

TOOLBOX

Seriously ask yourself if you can be happy with your body as it is.
If you can love it and live with it boldly and joyfully, do it!! You will save yourself a ton of grief and a whole lot of hassle. Stay healthy, strong, and strut your stuff. Let go of the whole pursuit of weight loss. It will be a huge relief.

If you do want to change, first decide which habits you are not ready to let go of.
Be specific. Take them off the table, and release yourself from any guilt associated with them.

Choose a few tips from this chapter, and give them a whirl.
The most powerful in my experience are: don't eat in front of the TV; go to bed earlier (and stop eating at least two hours before you do); and reduce your idea of what a portion size looks like. But feel each option out for yourself. See which are manageable and which make you feel better right off the bat.

Part III

Making It Last

The world will keep on turning without you burning out the gears
Seconds still collecting into just another year . . .
Lay back and let your mind get softer for a while.
We can let them fight for inches while we coast another mile . . .
I'm only hoping for a whole new state of mind,
a brand new paradigm.
> —Sons of Bill, Wilson, Abe. "Brand New Paradigm." Sons of Bill,
> *Love and Logic*, 2014

10

MINDFULNESS AND MINDLESSNESS

Several years into my career as a trainer, I was still eating at night to ease common anxiety and pass the time. It smoothed over the rough edges and filled me with disgust almost immediately afterward. I felt like I should be some sort of paragon of fitness and held myself to even higher standards than I had before. I might as well have weighed 300 pounds when, in fact, I was only 140. The mirror in my bathroom had a funhouse effect, bending and warping, depending on my frame of mind.

I ate pretty well during the days and was hiking and lifting weights regularly, but nights were almost always lost to mindless grazing. I was weary each morning, waking up to the knowledge that I had eaten uncontrollably the night before, and apprehensive as the sun went down, knowing that I would inevitably give in again, no matter how hard I tried to keep my impulses at bay.

The "decision" to relinquish control at night seemed to take place without my consent, and I couldn't understand why it was so hard to stop. I wasn't in crisis. I was just stressed out about the regular stuff of life, and food eased the disquiet. It allowed me to step out of my mind for an hour or two, until the following morning when regret surfaced, amplifying already palpable stress.

I desperately wanted to break free of the pattern. I was uneasy in my body *every day* because of what was happening at night, paying a heavy price for that fleeting relief. So I decided one day to take it on like Max takes on the monsters in Maurice Sendak's *Where the Wild Things Are*. "And Max said, 'BE STILL!' and tamed them with a magic trick of staring into all their yellow eyes without blinking once, and they were frightened and called him the wildest thing of all."[1]

I set my objective and steeled myself to stare directly into the yellow eyes of mindless eating, to bulldoze my way through. However many nights it took to come up against the worst of that powerful urge, I was determined to face it without giving in. I wanted to know if I could do it and what would happen on the other side.

The first day was relatively uneventful. I ate three meals with normal portion sizes and a few healthy snacks. I took deep breaths; kept myself busy with chores at night; and went to bed early, victorious. My stomach felt better already, and I got cocky heading into day two.

That second day, I made it through dinner and a few hours beyond, before familiar anxiety began cropping up. I stared at the TV and changed the channel. I paced the floor and thumbed through a book, but nothing could hold my attention. Around 10 p.m., I got a sinking feeling as panic seeped in through my chest like rising water in a flood. My eyes darted toward the kitchen.

I didn't have anything particularly succulent in the house, but there's always a way to satisfy that sugary, carby craving. I could make French toast; oatmeal with brown sugar; or the ultimate release: peanut butter chocolate chip cookie dough. I had all the tricks I craved behind the doors of those cabinets and none of the resolve to resist them.

I watched as my body stood up, and my feet moved through the tiny apartment toward the refrigerator, only a few steps between me and the entrance to the kitchen. I put my hand out to stop my body at the doorjamb; leaned against the wall; and sank to the floor—one butt cheek on the industrial living room carpet and the other on the yellowed linoleum of the kitchen floor—thirsting for the relief of a sugar coma.

I wrapped my arms around my knees and curled into the tightest ball I could build, trying to keep myself from crossing the threshold into the kitchen. I put my head between my hands and cried for cookie dough. I cried for the hundreds of times this had happened before and the hundreds of times I gave in; and I cried because I realized that I didn't know who I was if I wasn't someone who turned to food for comfort. Without that identity and all that came with it, I felt faceless, disoriented, and adrift.

In spite of all rational thought telling me I could be someone not addicted to food, I had no idea who that person might be or how she might handle anxiety without a fix to help her through. I slipped down the rabbit hole, and it was all I could do to stay put.

I sat there for what seemed like an hour, crying, pulling back and forth, leaning into and out of the kitchen, glued to the floor. Finally, exhausted, I pulled myself up, washed my face, and crawled into bed without eating a thing. I wanted to give in like always, of course, and forget the whole experiment, but so much more than that, on this night, I needed to confirm for myself that I could survive without turning to food, at least once. I wanted to remember what it was like to wake up without feeling defeated.

I got through the night and woke up in the morning, still alive, having discovered that what lay on the other side of my impulse to eat was nothing more and nothing less than a giant, heavy slab of emotion. It wasn't comfortable. In fact, it was miserable, but it wasn't going to *kill me* either—and this was a useful piece of information.

Staring down my own vulnerability was not going to kill me. It might make me *very* uncomfortable, but no matter how hard it got, I could survive it. It was a mass of yuck, and I could see why I preferred to avoid it most nights. But down on the kitchen floor, it was there and I was there, and I was able, for the first time, to see it plainly.

The American Buddhist nun, Pema Chödrön, wrote, "The most precious opportunity presents itself when we come to the place where we think we can't handle whatever is happening . . . you have no choice except to embrace [it] or push it away. . . . We use all kinds of ways to escape—all addictions stem from this moment when we meet our edge and we just can't stand it. . . . We become addicted to whatever it is that seems to ease the pain."[2]

I began to see that edge for what it was, difficult but not lethal. It was identifiable, and if it was identifiable, on some level, it was manageable. I could embrace it and live through it rather than always pushing it away with gobs of sweetness.

I wouldn't be able to muscle through like that for the long haul. It was too hard and unnatural to be sustainable, but I learned that I did possess the ability to make a different decision. It was possible. I survived being the crazy lady crying for cookie dough on the kitchen floor and woke up the next day, humbled but empowered.

Mindless eating always looks odd in the morning light. It's hard to remember why it even happens in the first place. It seems so obvious that it would have been better to make a different decision, but in the blur of the moment, it's difficult to give a damn. Diets will tell you what and when to eat, how and where to exercise, but in order to implement those plans, you have to get a handle on the blur.

One minute you're doing great and the next thing you know you're staring at yourself in the bathroom mirror with dark circles under your eyes and crusty crap plastered to your face. What happened? It's the blur, Lothario's spell, a wave of deep unconsciousness that overtakes you.

There are plenty of external ways to stop the onset of the blur. You can snap a rubber band around your wrist, eat an ice cube, do a handstand against the wall, hang upside down off of the couch—anything to jolt your brain and interrupt the momentum. The point is to sharpen your awareness and reel your thoughts back in—away from sources of anxiety and the intoxicating balm of your poison—to the present moment and the difficult decision right in front of you: To eat, or not to eat? To skip the workout, or show up and give it a go? What are your options?

When you wake yourself up like that, it's a greeting. *Hello! Welcome back to reality.* Welcome back to the same old decision. Does this thing lighten your load or weigh you down? How about trying something new this time so you don't have to feel like ass-crackers in the morning?

What we're really talking about is *mindfulness*, but that word is tossed around too easily, like we're all supposed to understand what it means. It sounds nice, but it's confusing too. Vague. Does it mean we're all supposed to meditate? Go to yoga? It's a pretty word, but how does it actually help?!

Mindfulness is a deep breath before placing your lunch order. It's a fully conscious moment before deciding whether to turn left toward home or right toward the trailhead. That's all. Not a big deal in and of itself. It's a step out of the pandemonium that allows for perspective, a visit with the "witness" I mentioned in chapter 3.

Think of it like the feeling you might get if you found a wallet on the street with hundreds of dollars in it. There's a hiccup in the moment when you realize the choice in front of you. You know the right and wrong thing to do. Pretty quickly, most of us would probably decide to look at the ID and return the wallet, but that breath before the decision is mindfulness. It's not necessarily an easy decision to make, but we do it anyway because we know which option will allow us to be at peace and feel good about ourselves. To take the money and toss the wallet would feel wrong. If we can apply that same principle to food and exercise, we go a long way toward making significant changes in our bodies.

To skip the walk or eat the extra egg roll feels just a little bit wrong, and we know it.

Making mindful decisions takes practice like anything else, but if you pay attention to how often the choice pops up between taking care and doing damage, you'll see how many opportunities there are to have a positive impact. Some impulses are hard to interrupt, but others aren't. Start by making the easiest choices first, staying conscious of taking better care a little at a time. Once you're doing that with relative ease, even if tougher decisions go down in flames, you're still doing better than you were before.

No new skill is ever effortless or flawless. It takes a while to learn to drive or play piano. Mastering anything you've never done before feels clumsy at the beginning but gets easier over time. The same can be said for mindfulness. You're learning how to pump the brakes instead of slamming them on and spinning out.

It feels halting and a little crazy at first to be standing in the cookie aisle at the grocery store silently counting to five before tossing the Chips Ahoy! into your cart. I used to shake my head like a wet dog before pulling into a drive-through in the middle of the afternoon. I got a lot of strange looks through the car window but also dodged a lot of calories and bloating that way. It starts with *one* time, one breath, and one decision to do something different. The first time is the hardest, but it continues to feel strange and untested as you move through decisions that were previously unconscious.

In the thickest part of the blur that night in my apartment, I stayed aware of the encroaching anxiety and the potent urge to eat. I was aware of my body moving through space toward the kitchen. I understood that I was anxious but not physically hungry, and I applied the brakes just enough to halt my body at the threshold. Whether I succeeded in making a better choice that night or not, the mindfulness, in and of itself, would have been a win.

The goal wasn't to transform my whole approach to food overnight. I just wanted to know I could stop the momentum. With that one victory, I learned that I was capable of paying attention to what was happening as it was happening and turning off the autopilot.

That level of vigilant awareness is intense and exhausting. It can't be sustained all the time and takes a while before it gets easier. In the process of working with it, I needed patience for it to become second nature and compassion for all the times the process would fall flat.

I returned to my cherished, cookie dough comfort zone many times in the following months. Sometimes I was able to make better decisions, but much of the time, I wasn't. It didn't matter, though. I was practicing and getting more adept at interrupting thoughtless impulses. When the desire for cookie dough came up, even if I chose to dive in, I was aware that *I had a choice* and made it consciously, which was worlds better than feeling out of control. The decision about whether to indulge or not became mine. I owned it, and once I did that, I was far more capable of making healthy decisions.

Greater awareness also gave me enough distance from the situation to see clearly that beating myself up for bad decisions only increased my likelihood of making *more* bad ones—and I certainly didn't want that. The only other option I had was to give it a break. Once I relaxed and let bad decisions float away as irreversible and forgivable, the balance began to tip. Peace with my body was on the horizon. I could taste it and thirst for it.

My standard-issue reasons for wanting to lose weight in the first place began to look shortsighted and irrational: weddings, reunions, date nights, beach trips. All of those things passed by and were over, seemingly, before they began. They were fleeting and not substantial enough to motivate me for the long term. I finally realized that the only reason good enough to choose salad over French fries was that salad made me feel better. I could think more clearly and handle stress better, breathe deeper, and jump higher if I wasn't weighed down by a bunch of fat and salt. Duh.

I finally recognized that the addiction was perpetuating itself. Eating too much for the wrong reasons made me feel *worse*, body and soul, not better—which made me want to eat again. Round and round. I wanted to be liberated, and the only way to do that was to interrupt the onset of the blur as it descended, to practice mindfulness like I was learning to drive—one careful turn, one wide-awake moment at a time.

About a year after the kitchen incident, in one of my shining moments on a particularly rough day, I stopped at the grocery store for some white cake mix and two tubs of fudge icing. I made a sheet cake for dinner in a 9 by 13-inch pan, cooled it in the freezer, iced it, and sat down in front of the TV with a giant bottle of club soda and a fork.

I knew what I was doing and decided I was fine with it. I took note of the weird, petroleum-like, waxy film building up on my lips and watched reality show contestants dashing through exotic foreign lands. I wasn't particularly sad or angry. I was a little numb, of course, but ate the cake consciously. I stayed aware of how it tasted; how it felt going into my stomach; how the dopamine in my brain surged; and how the sugar rush brought a deep sense of calm followed by a headache. I understood fully what was happening—and did it anyway.

Revisiting toxic, old patterns like that has proved helpful for me when I'm finally, just about ready to let them go. It eases an inner longing and reminds me how and why I feel crappy indulging like that. Sometimes a girl just needs to sit down and eat a cake in solitude.

The next day I chose not to punish myself. I didn't exercise for hours or starve myself. I knew that the best thing I could do was have a normal day with a nice, long walk; as much healthy, whole, satisfying food as I could scrounge up; and regular meetings with clients.

I met a new one that afternoon, named Laura, who came to me for fitness counseling. She booked the time a few days earlier, saying that her body ached and she couldn't find an exercise routine that felt right. She said she was jumbled up in her head and needed someone to help her sort out what to do next. She didn't tell me her age or body type over the phone, and when she showed up at my door, I was surprised. I expected an older woman in deteriorating condition, but in walked a twenty-five-year-old blonde, approximately five foot five, 110 pounds.

She told me she had struggled with body image since the age of eleven with the worst the fixation coming in her late teens and early twenties. She was hyper-aware of what she ate in social situations and fixated on the "bulges" on her belly and thighs. She wasn't comfortable enough to change clothes in front of other women in the locker room at the gym. She was newly married and didn't even want her husband to see her naked in a fully lit room because she felt "fat and ugly." She had a body any rational person would be thrilled to have, but her mind was too riddled with bullet holes and cheap shots to see it. She was slim, yes, but painfully self-conscious and insecure.

Laura is one of many examples I could give of people's insides not matching their outsides. Suffice it to say that, after thirteen years as a trainer, I have learned all too well that fit people do not have a monopoly on self-acceptance or confidence. Pretty much everyone subjects his or her body to scrutiny, and they are all imperfect. They're unique and smelly and loud and lumpy, but our only real option is to love them anyway—just as we consistently love and care for our friends' and families' bodies whether they are strong or weak. Going into combat with ourselves doesn't help, no matter what size we are. It only makes things worse.

Laura had a long road in front of her to ease up on the unnecessary pain she was inflicting on herself. She was entrenched in a critical mindset, shaming her body and robbing herself of pleasure. But she also had something powerful going for her. She could see that her approach was doing more damage than good. She was making an effort to stay conscious, mindful, and inquisitive. She was putting on the emergency brake, stepping back, and looking for perspective.

I wanted to wrap her up and take the pain away. She was stuck in her head, staring intently at the funhouse mirror, and looking to me to say something to fix it. I would have given the world to do it for her. She was searching, and I knew a thing or two about that search. But the truth was that I ate a cake the night before because I was lonely and stressed out. So I told her the only thing I could.

It's okay.

It's okay that you're self-conscious and stuck in your head, and it's okay that you feel "fat and ugly." But resenting yourself for being messed up won't make it any better. All you can do is recognize that you're looking in the wrong direction at the wrong thing. It's not about weight loss; it's about strength. Shift your focus; and *do something* tangible that makes you stronger and clearer today, and tomorrow, and the next day. Eventually your head will catch up. You'll be able to see more clearly that striving for wellness instead of "skinniness" can diminish the control that destructive thoughts and actions have over you—and a strong, slim, energetic body can develop from there. It's okay to feel like a mess. Let it be that way. Just add something new and healthy to the mix every chance you get, and keep moving in the right general direction.

Talking to her made me feel old, in a stable, wonderful kind of way. I waved as she walked out the door, back to her husband and the clutter filling her mind. For all intents and purposes, I was the teacher that day and she was the student—but, in fact, she taught me.

She reminded me how disconnected I had been from my body just a few years earlier; how much I had despised it; and how that hatred had driven me to stuff, starve, and manipulate it. As we sat in my living room, I saw from a distance the cavernous gap between the impossible, misery-inducing ideal I had been grasping at and the liberty I was now achieving.

I wasn't in my "ideal" weight range yet, and I had a cake for dinner the night before, but neither of those things mattered. I understood that it was a night and a cake, not the end of the world, and I had all the nights for the rest of my life to find a healthier way to calm my nerves. I woke up that morning with compassion in my heart for the sneaky, frightened little part of myself that got away with murder the night before, and let the body rest in peace.

It was mercy and freedom.

The condemnation was lifting, and Laura reminded me, in stark terms, how far I had come and how little I intended to go back.

Mindfulness breeds compassion by disarming hatred. It allows for a safe distance where there's nothing to lash out against and clearheaded decisions can prevail. It's not easy at first to remember to keep coming back to it. It takes effort to step away in your mind; see what's happening; and not pass judgment on it—but with practice, that pause begins to bring relief, and remembering to stop (and reassess) gets easier.

In the thick of the blur, mindfulness allows you to actually *implement* the healthy living directives you find in this and other wellness books. It turns off your autopilot and frees you to make decisions that will serve your body and mind.

The scariest, most detrimental place to be is in a state of unconsciousness—perpetuating destructive behavior repeatedly and checking out while you do it. Instead of fighting that behavior, just notice it. See the situation for what it is. Notice the boredom or sadness as it rises and triggers the desire to head for the fridge. Notice the compulsive thoughts fixating on pizza. Eat it if you must, but *own* that decision instead of blocking it out. Satiate the impulse in the short term, knowing it will burrow down and resurface again later, whining and crying out again for a cheesy deluxe at midnight.

When it does, if you own it again and face it again, each time it comes back up, whether you overcome it or give into it, it will be weaker, wielding less power over you because you will have called it out, not merely responded to it unconsciously. Eventually, you'll get bored and annoyed by the same old, destructive siren call, and you'll be prepared to make a different decision.

Whatever you do, don't check out. Staying conscious, you'll come to know in your heart and body that food is not the solver of all problems. A bucket of fried chicken will not make your boss back off, and pint of ice cream will not keep you company. They will try, but they will fail.

Every mindful moment is a success. If it leads to a healthy decision, bonus. At the beginning, just stay present in whatever dose you can manage. Look for the moment when your best judgment begins washing away, and halt it before deciding what to do one way or the other. That's where it starts.

Beyond mindfulness is *mindlessness*, and that's where the payoff really begins—when mindfulness isn't all that necessary anymore because you're too busy being present, enjoying your life and body just as they are.

Mindlessness is a concept lost on most of us born and raised in the western hemisphere. We think it's a negative thing. We translate it as thoughtlessness or disregard for things that matter, but I see it as just the opposite. Mindlessness, to me, is the poignancy of holding your grandmother's hands in yours as her fingers tremble with age. It's the astonishment and terror of holding a newborn baby in your arms; or the quiet that comes when you sit at the edge of the water with your favorite companion at your side. There's nothing to say, nothing to think, not a single word that could illuminate the experience beyond the simple living of it.

Mindlessness is the closest we get to eternity, and when it comes to our bodies and the seemingly endless dialogue we engage in about what we should or shouldn't be doing, it is a living luxury to simply be inside of them, to appreciate them and mindlessly take better care of them because it feels right—to order a glass of water instead of a soda without any internal debate, to wander around the neighborhood because it feels nicer than sitting in the house staring at a computer screen.

Mindfulness halts the flow of destructive moments.

Mindlessness is when you get to be free of the whole thing.

For control freaks like myself, the easiest way to practice that blissful release is to rely heavily on the infrastructure that holds my health and sanity together, whatever comes my way to have unshakeable knowledge of (and faith in) the steel bars at the center of my pod. With that in place, it's remarkably easy to make the best decisions I can and let the rest go.

I need to walk and hike. I need access to sunshine and air, time spent curled up with furry animals, and regular contact with my soul shine people. I need clients to remind me that strength comes in every shape and size. With any or all of those things in place, I can ride the wave of whatever else starts to go awry.

It doesn't matter what your personal support beams are, as long as you know them as intimately as you know your own name. They might even include a deliciously wonderful, old, bad habit that can keep you stable while you work out the other, new ones. If you can remember to lean on those beams in times of need, you will find yourself free to be mindless more often than not, with no threat at all to your well-being. When something starts feeling wrong or careening out of control (which it always, eventually does), be mindful of the disconnect and turn—without hesitation—back to your infrastructure for support.

You are creating *one* process of growth that can stand up whether you're in crisis or celebration. That bedrock response and the tools at your disposal are always the same. They will continue moving you toward better and away from worse, regardless what obstacles arise. The beams you choose will create and grow the environment around you, and that environment will begin to hold you up. It will allow space, treasured, amazing space, for mindlessness.

We know that food (sugar, in particular) triggers the same parts of the brain as drugs,[3] but research is showing that addiction isn't simply the result of chemical dependence. Isolation and stress play a huge part in addictive behavior as well. The environment we live in, the connections we have with others, and the contributions we make at home and work strongly impact how susceptible we are to dependence.

The British journalist Johann Hari spent years researching and writing a book about the causes of addiction.[4] He wrote an article about it for *Huffington Post*, called "The Likely Cause of Addiction Has Been Discovered, and It Is Not What You Think," outlining two studies that prove the point.[5] In the first study he describes, it's estimated that 20 percent of Vietnam War veterans were addicted to heroin while overseas at war, but after returning home to healthy environments, 95 percent of them "simply stopped" using it, with little to no intervention. This is in stark contrast to addiction relapse rates estimated as high as 90 percent in the general public, depending which research you're looking at.[6]

In the second study, rats given access to cocaine-laced water drank themselves to death if left alone in drab cages, but after being placed into stimulating rat playgrounds with a community of friends and family, they dropped the habit by choice with very few withdrawal symptoms.

"It isn't you. It's your cage," Hari writes.

Addiction of any kind is frightening and complex with many physiological drivers. Clearly anyone who needs support with addiction should seek professional help,[7] but Hari's work illuminates a truth I have seen time and again with my clients. As their lives grow more engaging and rewarding, as they root out causes of stress and replace them with sources of fulfillment, they are drastically less likely to turn to food in search of relief and much more likely to reach their fitness goals.

Know what works for you. Have a ready list of healthy habits to turn to. Figure out new ways to connect with friends and colleagues, and help out somebody in need whenever you possibly can. Rely on those things. With a support structure like that in place, mindfulness can help you remember that you have a choice about how to proceed in any given moment. And mindlessness is the reward. Hours that stretch into weeks, months, and finally years, easy in your skin with a quiet, innate sense of how much is too much and how much isn't enough.

TOOLBOX

Practice mindfulness like any other skill.

There are a million ways to regain awareness when you find yourself going off the rails. I mentioned a few earlier: snap a rubber band around your wrist, eat an ice cube, hang upside down, shake your head vigorously, chew gum, or brush your teeth. I've known people who smell vanilla extract or drink a glass of water every time they have a sugar craving. Do ten jumping jacks, juggle, snap your fingers, recite a favorite poem in your head, or sit down with your cat on the floor for a minute. It doesn't matter what it is as long as it's easy and it can interrupt the onset of your bad habit quickly enough for you to recognize the situation and make a conscious decision about whether or not to proceed.

Those are useful tricks, but if you want to dig deeper to unseat the impulses at their root, try meditation. A lot of people are intimidated by it and understandably so, but it doesn't need to be complicated or time-consuming. It's really just a dedicated practice for recognizing thoughts and habits as they come up and letting them drift off again without doing any damage. It creates a central, still, nonjudgmental place where there's no reason to be reactionary. It allows you to get comfortable with discomfort so you don't feel the urgent need to medicate it with your regular fix.

Spend a few minutes every day, sitting in a comfortable position, watching your thoughts ebb and flow. Here they come; there they go. When you find yourself thinking or worrying about them, just acknowledge them and bring your attention back to your breath. And then do it again with the next irritating thought. Start with as little as two or three minutes if that's all you have time for, but, if possible, do it every day. It needs to be practiced like anything else.

It might feel like nothing at first, and that's fine. You aren't likely to start levitating and emanating light from your crown chakra any time soon. Just think of it as a few minutes of release. If you don't want to sit, you can do it walking or washing dishes or doing any other repetitive activity. Just come back to your breath. Every nasty, happy, or heartbreaking thought can come and go, and your body will still be there, breathing you forward. Thoughts are just thoughts. You don't have to buy into each and every one.

To apply it directly to food and exercise, come back to those conscious breaths before placing a food order, before digging in to a meal, or halfway through to reassess how hungry (or not hungry) you are. Do it on the treadmill before deciding whether or not to press on, or in the car when deciding whether or not to go to the gym in the first place.

See the Further Readings list at the end of the book for more meditation resources.

Treasure mindlessness.

In addition to being mindful, take a few minutes of every day to step away from all of your distractions with something or someone (or in a place) that gives you aimless, thoughtless, simple, genuine peace. Just be there, breathe it in, and be thankful. At least once a day.

On top of that, recall healthy changes you've made in the past that are now second nature. The best ones are so engrained in your regular routine that you forgot you used to live without them. Did you used to drink soda for breakfast? Did you used to be grossed out by whole grain bread but now you love it? Did you used to be totally inactive but now you have a dog and go walking once a day? Did you used to get winded running for one minute, but now you can go for ten?

Notice those changes again, how mindless and easy they are now, and realize that other, new habits will eventually be just as easy if you keep reinforcing them.

Last, *give* mindlessly whenever possible and without expectation. See how effortless it is. Hand out compliments freely. Smile at strangers. Lend a hand. Check up on somebody. It doesn't cost a dime, but it will reveal a whole lot more clear, blue sky.

Forgive your bad habits.

What do you beat yourself up for? Eating at night, like me? Coffee and chocolate every day at 3 p.m.? Haven't exercised in months? It is what it is. There's no erasing it, so give yourself a break. Put your focus on what you can do right now, today, and go do it. Forward ho.

Revisit your infrastructure.

By now, you should have a pretty good idea of which habits you love that also keep you healthy. Make a solid list in your mind or journal. Short and sweet. Three or four things you can rely on—always, no matter what—to help you keep your universe together. Know them, love them, and lean on them for the rest of your life.

Take a look at your cage.

As you practice mindfulness, see if there are any constants associated with bad food or exercise habits. Are you generally in the same place or with the same people when bad habits kick in? Are you in a foul mood due to some sort of recurring situation? Move the couch. Disconnect the cable. Ask to be transferred to a different job with a different supervisor. Find a new school for your kid. Move. Break up with your boyfriend. Propose to your boyfriend. Learn to dive.

Have a look at what is pulling you under, and be inventive about how to break free. Concoct a harebrained scheme. It might not look so crazy if you think about it for a while, or it might lead to other ideas. Whatever you do, don't sit passively in your cage wondering why you can't stop reaching for food to keep you placated. Use mindfulness to implement tangible changes.

11

STARTING WHERE YOU ARE

My friend and client Elizabeth is a troubadour. A forty-five-year-old blues singer from Alabama, she is tall with long dark hair, happily married with a five-year-old son. She speaks Italian fluently and spent years of her early adult life living in Sweden and Italy. She has known many lovers and lost two of them, one to suicide, the other to substance abuse. She has been a model, a Harley-Davidson mechanic, and a chandelier maker. She maintains dear friendships in cities around the world where she has crooned her way into the hearts of audiences, and the players who accompany her on stage revere her for the chanteuse that she is. She has a killer life.

Elizabeth also happens to weigh four hundred pounds.

She is a paradox, a living, walking definition of both vitality and dysfunction. Her body is a burden; there's no way around it. But it's also the vehicle by which she has lived an exciting, glamorous life. She has never been small, and food and exercise have never been easy. She has clear memories of her mom being "ecstatic" when she decided to stop eating at age twelve and go on a liquid diet. Throughout her childhood, Elizabeth's portions were rationed at family dinners while everyone else ate their fill. Her friends gave her laxatives, and doctors gave her Fen-Phen (diet pills that were later banned for causing lethal heart problems).

"My genes are on the big side," she says, "I've always been bigger than average, but growing up into that hyper-controlling environment was the worst thing that could have happened. If I had just been left alone, I probably would have been fine. I certainly wouldn't have been this big.

"Problem is, it all became *my* doing at some point. I took the voices into my own head. I mean, I kept eating because I was so mad at myself for all the stupid shit I did—gaining weight and whatever else. I punished myself, but what's funny is, at this point I've let myself off the hook. I don't even care anymore who is judging me, but now here I am in this body. It's a whole other level of frustration. I did this. It's done, and I'm over beating myself up about it, but now, holy crap, this weight is heavy to lift. The hardest thing is that I *want* to move more. I want to be around for my kid. I want to be strong and healthy, but if I go out for a thirty-minute walk, it's so exhausting; it takes hours to recover from it. With food, I eat pretty healthy. I don't make terrible choices. I just have too much. But I'm not trying to make drastic changes any more. I just need to move more and eat a little less."

When she's not forcing herself into thirty-minute hill walks, Elizabeth is energetic and irreverent. She is an endless source of mindboggling stories and one of the kindest, most open people I've ever had the pleasure of knowing, but she has struggled with obesity, thyroid problems, and ankle and foot injuries her whole life.

When I met her for the first time, I watched as she moved carefully through the room and sat down with the aid of her arms. She told me everything she had been through with her weight over the years: when she lost and gained, and all of the underlying ups and downs in her life that precipitated those changes. She had trainers off and on and lost some weight with various diet programs. Five years before we met, she lost seventy-five pounds and planned a trip to Europe to celebrate, play a few shows, and see some friends. But when she boarded the plane, she discovered that, even after all her hard work, the seat belt still wouldn't fit around her abdomen. She asked for a seat belt extender and spent the eight-hour, transatlantic flight mulling over how pointless the whole effort had been. Losing weight was a constant battle, and here in her lap was proof that she was still huge. Her newly acquired perception of herself as thin (or at least, thinner) collapsed. What remained was the same old fat girl she knew so well, squeezed into a coach seat, asking for a plus-sized safety device. The whole thing was too taxing to not have made "any difference," so she surrendered all of her hard work to the black nylon webbing of the seat belt extender.

It didn't matter in that moment that she felt better than she had in years. She made the mistake of measuring her progress by the length of that belt rather than by how she felt. If she had used that time on the plane to think about how much more comfortable the seat was than ever before; or how much easier it was to get from the ticket counter to the gate; or how, after landing, she could walk easily from ancient ruins to a pub to a concert hall; she would have realized that the seat belt extender was irrelevant.

After the trip, she arrived home defeated. Soon after that, her beloved eleven-year-old puppy died. Then she injured her ankle and was unable to walk normally for months. The weight came pouring back on, and then some.

Here's the hard truth: Elizabeth will likely never be able to lose hundreds of pounds and keep it off with sheer determination and willpower by following all "the rules." It would be too miserable of an existence, and it would take *way* too long for her to feel like she has arrived at her happy place.

If she tries to do *everything right!* for months and years on end, that falsely enthusiastic, straight and narrow path will lead her, eventually, to want to claw her eyeballs out with a melon scooper. There's too much fire in her. There's no way she won't rebel against a life full of constraints. She'll get lost in a maze of supplements and elliptical machines, calorie counters and fat grams, and finally, simply say *screw it*. Again.

Unfortunately, science is not on her side either. Figuring out how to overcome lifelong obesity is one of the most perplexing problems of modern biology. A study by the *International Journal of Obesity* shows that, in overweight people who have consumed a high-fat diet for extended periods of time, the chemical and neurological signals from the stomach that kick in to tell them they're full are not working properly anymore; and the problem persists even after those people have changed their diets and lost weight. [1]

Deep breath. I know that sounds discouraging, but it's actually not the end of the world. They're saying that changing just long enough to lose the weight won't solve the problem. We knew that already. The changes have to be enduring and lifelong, but maintaining them isn't so difficult if you come at it from the right angle, if every step is laced with a little bit of pleasure. I don't want to blow smoke here. It's hard, really hard to lose weight and keep it off, but knowledge is power. With your focus on steady, healthy indulgences that stem from your interests, you'll have every reason to keep going no matter how long or slow the process of finding your featherweight body might be.

For Elizabeth, the messages from her brain to stop eating may not ever kick in as early as they would for other people, and if her brain and stomach aren't connecting right, she can't rely on them to guide her. She may never get the feeling of satiety that the rest of us achieve with appropriate portion sizes, and if that's the case, it's a loss worth mourning. She has an extra hurdle to jump, but knowing that gives her a whole hell of a lot more leverage than she had before. If she understands that her brain will consistently tell her to eat more than she needs, she has a fighting chance of doing something about it.

There's a middle ground between hunger and satisfaction that *anybody* who wants to eat less without feeling deprived needs to get intimate with. It happens about halfway through a meal when you're no longer starving but want to keep eating. Most people blow right past it, but if Elizabeth can find peace and familiarity with the sensation of being "not hungry" rather than with being "satisfied," she can make a dedicated practice of *quenching her hunger* rather than eating until she's full. It's actually a pretty nice feeling to be "not hungry." It's certainly better than feeling stuffed and weighed down. If she can do that, most or at least part of the time, she will make a huge dent in her calorie intake and lose weight. When she does eat to full satisfaction, which can happen as often or infrequently as she chooses, she can savor it.

Food is an offering for your body. When you start paying attention to when that feeling of genuine hunger passes, you'll be amazed how much less food you actually need. I've done it myself, and then I forget, and then I remember. But when I remember, I am infinitely lighter and never, ever hungry.

To move from being morbidly obese to being plain-old-regular obese to being average, Elizabeth has to make a seismic shift. The end goal is so far away from the present reality that it seems untouchable, so the payoff for making positive changes has to be moved into the present. What she's shooting for has to be immediate, and the way she measures success has to be based on what she can achieve *right now*. She has to learn anew how to receive and interpret the messages her body is sending—and translate them into routines that both lighten her step and keep her sane in the present, not in some vague, undetermined, fantasy future.

This is easily illustrated by her story because of the enormous task she faces, but it applies to anybody facing an uphill battle trying to get in shape.

If the changes she makes feel good right away and the rewards she gets resonate in a way that makes her feel like she is nurturing her vitality—if she senses that life-giving shift in her bones and under her skin—no seat belt extender will ever throw her off again. It might send her spinning out into the blur for a day or two, but it won't be enough to divert her for the long haul because continuing on will feel so much better than giving up.

A thirty-minute walk is too big of a task to begin with for her, but five or ten minutes isn't. Consistently parking as far as possible from the store entrance isn't. Ordering her enchiladas with red sauce instead of cheese sauce isn't. There are a million small things she can do that can make a big difference when pulled together.

She's already set up for success because she's finished beating herself up. All she wants to do is take better care so life starts feeling easier, and that is an extraordinary and peaceful place to begin. She's ready to start where she is and do what feels good. In my experience, that's closer to clarity and freedom than many people ever get.

Her thyroid is under control. She has learned that she loves to swim which takes the pressure off of her joints. There's no physiological reason why she can't lose at least some of the weight if that's what she wants, but she *cannot* try to leap from four hundred to two hundred pounds in one magnificent, spontaneous push. Her brain has built behaviors and neural pathways that support her body and life as they are, and it takes time for those things to change. She has lost fifty to a hundred pounds many times in her life, but she did it based on deprivation. This time, finally, she's doing it right—by treating herself well.

If she walks ten minutes every day; swims once or twice a week; and eats portions that are 10 percent smaller than usual, she will lose weight—no question—and she will feel better, whether she gets down to 375 or 275. But even small changes like that can throw off her equilibrium in ways that could make her want to go running back to the status quo. So each change, every single one, should feel like progress, expansion, liberation. Eating 10 percent less will only stick when it feels like freedom to be lighter at the end of a meal.

Diets and fitness schemes mess us up because they are based on making us less of who we are. *Don't eat that food you love. Do this exercise you hate.* The whole approach doesn't make sense. It's truly backward, and it starts in adolescence, the very first time we identify the thickening of our bodies as a defect rather than a source of power, as we ready ourselves for the challenges of adulthood.

From there, we embark on a mission to shrink ourselves, to make our bodies smaller than they naturally are. We spend enormous energy controlling and depriving ourselves with no concept of how insane the pursuit has been from the very beginning. And then there is the backlash. All of that time and effort spent hacking away at our native bodies does nothing but send us ricocheting back to all the food we resented giving up in the first place. It backfires, and unnecessary, unwanted weight piles on.

Enough already.

Bodies are beautiful because of *what they can do*, not because of how tiny they are. It's easy to forget what matters: the ability to bound up a flight of stairs to share good news, or the ability to stand outside on a cool, fall evening watching a storm roll in, with legs and strong abdominals to hold you up; clear vision to see dark clouds over a gray sky; ears to hear the scrape of leaves blowing on the sidewalk; the smell of rain on the horizon; and a chill on your skin.

Elizabeth may be big, but she is also powerful. And she is ready to care for her body in a new way. The seeds of that transformation began with her pregnancy. Working with me, she had already lost forty pounds by eating better and exercising more when she discovered that she was pregnant. From that moment on, she focused on nourishing herself instead of losing weight. It sounds small, but the shift was monumental. She let her body take the lead, telling her when she was hungry and when it was time to rest. She took care of herself and her baby, and six weeks after giving birth, she weighed ten pounds *less* than before she got pregnant—a total weight loss of fifty pounds from supporting her body instead of working against it.

I wish I could say she kept that fifty pounds effortlessly off, but she wasn't ready yet. She needed one more ride on the merry-go-round to remind her that taking up arms against her body will never land her in a healthy place.

She got panicky about keeping it off and trying to lose more. Being a new mom is hard. She lost sleep, trying to make a living and being available for her family. She hated her job but slogged through a few more years before realizing that it was at the center of a downward spiral that was beginning to threaten her life. When the weight started coming back, it seemed like a foregone conclusion. She decided sugar was the culprit and quit it for a while before falling off of the wagon. Old cycles were back in force.

But the shock of new motherhood passed, and I've seen a different woman emerging recently. She quit her job and is squeaking out a living teaching Italian, renting out her basement as a vacation rental, and making music. She's gone back to her scrappy roots. I see the Harley-Davidson mechanic emerging again, and it's about time.

"I'm already seeing results from what I've done the last month," she says. "I'm stronger. I stand up from a chair, and I can feel my stomach muscles go in, pushing me up. That's improvement. My skin cleared up. My eyes are brighter. I've got some momentum. I don't feel like I'm having the soul sucked out of me every day. Moving is hard work, and it's going to stay hard for a while. But I can feel physical changes from what I'm doing. I'm feeling so much better and doing it all for that."

Elizabeth will always be bigger than most, but her delight in living is too great to continue to cripple herself with cumbersome, unmanageable body weight. Finally, after too many years, she recognizes that her body is an ally, not an enemy, and that the best thing she can do is treat it well. She is setting up an environment where she can thrive.

Quitting her job won't solve everything. Neither will meal planning or exercising. The hard truth is that she finds herself, today, in a four-hundred-pound body with a young son and a host of other challenges. She has a lot to deal with, but she is finished being pissed off. She's interested in being capable and functional, feeling whole and at peace.

Now that she's done brooding about her weight, she's free to take a stroll after dinner because it gives her time to write melodies in her head—and free to stop when she gets tired, leaving enough energy for the following day to continue moving and breathing. Those little walks are a radical reclamation of her lungs, and her lungs are the things that have always given her life. She's giving back to them now. Wherever she goes, whatever she does next, she will be singing, always singing, her voice a harbinger of things to come—a lighter life and a freer body.

I told Elizabeth's story recently to a young woman named Cora who is in the early years of her own journey with her body. She's a sophomore in college now, but I've known and worked with her since she was a junior in high school. In many ways, she's an average kid, but she was dealt a tough blow with regard to her health very early in life. With a little preemptive awareness, Cora has an extraordinary opportunity to develop a relationship with her body based on renewal rather than restraint.

When she was ten years old, an abnormal clump of veins on her brainstem called an AVM hemorrhaged and caused her to have a stroke while playing on the beach with her parents. She underwent four surgeries over the following eight years to correct the problem. Until the last surgery, her body and brain were functioning normally, except for some mild numbness in her limbs.

Cora spent the entirety of her teenage years under the watchful eye of doctors and parents. Her health and well-being were of concern to everyone around her. She did her best to care for her body as she grew through the awkwardness of puberty, but the vigilance expected of her was a heavy lift for a little kid.

She began gaining weight after the first surgery at eleven years old, due to medication and extended stays in the hospital. Bullied and unhappy in school, she gained more in junior high, and her weight became a pressing issue for her parents as they grew concerned that it would increase her blood pressure and the likelihood of another stroke.

When she gained another thirty pounds her junior year, their concern grew to alarm. They were terrified to lose her. In an attempt to help, her mom began feverishly fixating on Cora's nutrition and portion sizes. They limited her calories and examined the nutritional value of every morsel that passed through her lips. Her parents meant well. They are loving, educated people who, along with Cora, endured a terrifying ordeal, but their well-intended coaching fell on the ears of their ailing daughter like it would on the ears of any teenage girl.

When they said, "We're concerned about your weight," she heard, "You're fat, and it's not okay." The measured portion sizes began to feel like rationing; the daily inquisition about her eating habits made her overly conscious of food; and weekly weigh-ins inspired her to reach for laxatives.

Her entire adolescence felt beyond her control, and she desperately wanted that control back any way she could get it. By senior year, she was stealing money from her parents' wallets so she could cut out of school before lunch to inhale an entire box of cookies and a full-size bag of chips at the drugstore next door. Adults were always telling her what to eat and not to eat—but that pre-lunch binge was *her* time, one moment in her day when no one was watching and she could do whatever she wanted.

Two weeks before leaving for college, she mentioned her final surgery to me in one of our exercise sessions, almost as an afterthought to let me know that she needed to cancel our appointments the following week. Her doctors were optimistic that they could choke the AVM off with this last surgery, once and for all, and that she would be ready to leave for school with no problem.

But when she woke up from anesthesia, Cora had lost all sensation and coordination on the left side of her body. She was unable to walk without a cane and had no control over her left arm or hand. College was off the table for at least another year while she underwent intensive physical and occupational therapy to repair the damage. A clinic in New Mexico helped her walk again, and another in Louisiana got her left arm moving again, but left her with a severe and persistent tremor. It was arduous work, but she only had two choices. She could do everything in her power to get better, or give up. And she wasn't interested in giving up.

Between physical therapy intensives, she exercised with me and took classes at a local university in karate, silk screening, and poetry. She got a small apartment in student housing a few miles from her parents' home as part of the therapy to encourage independent living. With that little bit of freedom, her weight finally stopped rising.

Trying to find her way through the frustration of barely discernable progress, she dove in to worlds that stretched her identity, exploring tattoos and bisexuality. To her parents, she was a treasured but wild child; to me, she was the hope of the future, deeply emotional and as smart as they come. There was no doubt she was rebelling and medicating anxiety with food, but it wasn't the crisis they imagined. She just needed a little space and some tools to help her cope. She met with nutritionists and counselors and continued her sessions with me.

After a full year of rehab, the tremor remained in her left hand, and she never regained feeling on the left side of her body—but she could walk and write, date and draw. She pressed through the fear and adversity she faced to unearth whatever reinforcements she could find and to build the strongest, most functional body possible.

When finally preparing all over again for college, like any kid leaving home for the first time, Cora was ecstatic in anticipation of the freedom she would gain. She hoped that being discharged from all of those watchful eyes would release her from her rebellious urge to eat, but like Elizabeth, those voices were already making their way into her own mind.

Going forward, Cora has the unusual advantage of knowing intimately, far too young, that health is a precious commodity and that it is her responsibility and her life's work to take care of it in every way she can.

She's studying anthropology now with a focus on human sexuality and social justice, and she wrote an insightful article for the school newspaper about what it's like to function in the world, and in particular, to go on dates as a disabled person.

"It's so interesting to me," she says, "how we make snap judgments about people based on how they look, what race they are, or how much money they have. I'm an overweight, queer, white girl with a disability, but studying this stuff, I'm thinking about things in a different way. People live with disabilities all the time, and they're amazing. I might never be able to carry a tray and be a waitress, but that's cool. I really just want to unlearn all of the toxic assumptions I've internalized. I want to take care of myself. I exercise now because it makes me more 'with it' mentally. I sleep better too. I'm not doing it to lose weight. I'm doing it because it makes me feel good. I'm doing squats for me because it's amazing that I can, not because somebody else thinks I should."

Cora's plans have been shattered time and again: to have a normal childhood and adolescence and to leave for college intact and on time. Her struggles are obvious to the world. There is no hiding it. She can't feed herself with her left hand or hold a book like any of us might without shaking uncontrollably. But instead of letting her situation defeat her, she is allowing it to mold her into a thoughtful, intelligent adult who will have a great deal to say in the coming years about the plight of the disabled and disenfranchised.

She plans to get inked one day with an image of the AVM that forever altered the arc of her life and the state of her body. She'll wear it like a badge of honor. It has informed her and required her to develop coping skills that will serve her well as she encounters challenges that have nothing at all to do with numbness or tremors.

Cora has a long road in front of her, but so do the rest of us who are striving to build new, neural pathways; to strengthen our bodies; and increase balance and agility. Her path is harder, but the pursuit is the same. We should all hope to be so irrepressible. She has done, under incredibly trying circumstances, what all of us are capable of doing every day if we stay focused on the right objectives.

Life threw Cora a nasty curveball, and through everything that came along with that, she has dedicated herself to reconstructing a body that will carry her blithely through the rest of her life. She values her body for what it's capable of. Her social media feed boasts puffy, beautiful, lipstick-laden lips, the curve of her neck, the arc of a lover's back, and kick-ass glasses she got after being forbidden to wear contact lenses for fear she might scratch a cornea.

She looks for what works and is learning to claim her independence in ways that don't involve binging on junk food. She is allowing her body to inform her, to propel her forward and ground her in a version of herself that is overflowing with possibilities and ways to contribute. It's been a rough ride so far, but whatever she ends up doing, she plans to have a good time along the way. AVM be damned, her body is her own.

Cora and Elizabeth are both curious, unstoppable souls. They're fighters. Elizabeth picked an ill-fated fight with her weight when she was very young with no intention of surrendering, and I have seen Cora beginning to do the same.

Elizabeth's fight expanded into a full-blown battle, and the battle mushroomed into a war that has defined her life. She faces the consequences now and will spend the coming years clearing away wreckage to make peace with her body in her fifties, sixties, and beyond.

She has the wisdom of hindsight now and the calm compassion that comes with age, but she also faces profound regret that she put on so much weight by being unable to appreciate the incredible utility of her body sooner. The only way forward from here is to start moving in the right direction and keep on trekking. At forty-five, she's got half a lifetime left to live and finally understands that cherishing her body instead of fighting it is the only way to make it better.

Cora is twenty-one years old and thirty pounds heavier than she might like to be. If she can begin now to focus her fight on *bolstering* her body while sharpening her skills and mind, she will find herself at age forty-five in a body that supports her life—with or without the tremor. The number she sees on the scale will be an afterthought; and the shape of her hips and thighs a beautiful inheritance, a reflection of the women she sprang from, the life she has lived, and the food and exercise she has loved.

Bodies are beautiful because of their functionality and uniqueness. The fight to shrink and tuck them has been with us for far too long, and it has failed. The war is lost, and it is my fervent, idealistic hope that this living generation is the one that will step out of the fray and make it stop, that we are the ones who will finally prioritize nourishment and strength over appearance.

This movement is already taking hold with waves of body positive blogs and advertising campaigns, neighborhood gardens, community supported agriculture, makeup-free dolls and action figures for girls,[2] and elementary school nutrition and wellness education. Corporate culture is slowly awakening to the fact that lunchtime walks, access to healthy food, and on-site exercise facilities increase productivity and profits and decrease health insurance expenses.

I hope that upcoming generations will look back at the last fifty years of fad diets and plastic surgery with sadness and pity for the poor people who endured those bizarre expectations and wasted incalculable energy, time, and money trying to achieve weirdly homogenized and impossible ideals.

The greatest contribution we can make is to love and appreciate our bodies for the astonishing creations that they are, to feed them and move them in ways that bring them to life—one body at a time, one community at a time. Imagine the legacy we would pass to our children, especially our daughters, if they saw us stretching and stimulating our bodies, never starving or sucking in. Imagine what it would be like to walk through a world of people who care more about vitality, kindness, and insight than about pant size.

Cora's generation can do it. They are fearless, unapologetic, and raw, and if they continue to harness their energy for good, they have the potential to create a perfect storm. They're pushing boundaries in tech, innovation, and art. They believe that they have the right to speak out and to educate themselves (and eventually their children) in the way they see fit. As they grow into more influential roles, if they can persevere in sourcing their power from their intelligence and aptitude instead of their measurements, they can quietly create new assumptions about what success looks like. And it will look like fortitude, steadiness, and dexterity—at any size.

Elizabeth's generation, starting just as they are, can pave the way for those younger women by switching gears mid-life to realign their priorities with authentic wellness. It's a natural time for it. By forty, we have a lot of ties that bind, a lot of demands on our physical and mental energy. We have many things more valuable to think about than how our thighs look. I'm told that people tend to stop caring so much about what others think after age forty. I'm nearly there, and all signs are good so far. I wish it could have come sooner.

As smart, functional individuals, there's no good reason to apologize for the uniqueness of our bodies, and the only reason to change them is to help them become more vital and alive.

No matter how unfit you might be, no matter how old or young, the narrative can change from wherever you are. Your objective can switch from weight loss to strength, and strength can be built from the outside in. Old habits will die hard. The cow path is well tread. The cookie dough craving will endure, but if your mission is to fortify your body rather than strip it down, temporary obstacles won't stand a chance of throwing you off.

Start where you are, and take small steps toward new and different. It's about getting out in the sunshine and walking as many steps as possible because it's freeing; cultivating a taste for things that grow out of the earth because they taste alive; and rejecting things that grow out of a box because they taste like the cardboard they're packed in. It's about discovering when your heart and mind are craving solace, and finding a way, other than food, to meet that need. It's about building that one unified system to support one unique, exceptional body. It's about filling life with compelling stuff. Small, steady changes.

I ran into Elizabeth recently at our local pool. She stood in the shallow end in her bathing suit, playing with her son, wearing a straw hat and bright red sunglasses. She was surrounded by dozens of moms and twenty-somethings who were half her size, tugging at swimsuits and shielding themselves in oversized towels. With a nod and a knowing laugh, she shook her head. "I'm done," she said, "totally done."

I'm with Elizabeth. Done.

TOOLBOX

Utilize your body.

Your body serves you. It makes it possible for you to get to class or work and to care for the people you love. It makes it possible for you to hang out with your friends and throw back a few too many. Your body is on your side. When you find yourself beating up on it, *use it* for something useful to remind yourself how much value it holds: organize your space; plunk out a tune on the piano; or water your plants.

If you have two good legs, get up and walk. If you have two good arms, pick up a camera or some knitting needles and make something beautiful. Even without a fully functional body, you can make use of what you have. As Cora can attest, a lot of people can't see, drive, walk, or brush their hair, much less ride a bike or do a handstand. But people with disabilities accomplish incredible things all the time because they recognize the value of the capabilities they have left.

Make use of your body. Every move is remarkable, and if you can accomplish even more than the basic tasks of daily life, you are winning. Challenge that beautifully imperfect body to go just beyond your comfort zone to accomplish a new move or skill. Reclaim its usefulness.

Make positive changes that have nothing to do with diet and exercise.

Clean out your inbox; sign up for a cooking class; get a pet; get out of a damaging job, relationship, or living environment. Try volunteering. It will shift your focus from your own problems to helping somebody else with theirs. When you find yourself stressing about a body part or habit you don't like, busy your mind by thinking about how to wiggle out of one boring or frustrating situation, into a more rewarding one.

12

WIDE OPEN

I went dancing recently with a group of friends on a Friday night. Exhausted after a long week, we were unsure if our bodies, of all different shapes, would hold up for the long haul, but the retro pop swept us up. The smartest among us wore sneakers; the diehards sported heels. I split the difference in wedges and a turquoise tutu. After raising our arms to the ceiling for several hours and sweating like a pack of animals, we walked outside into the pouring rain, took off our shoes, and walked home, drenched in surrender.

"It's like church," I said, padding along in bare feet through the puddles. I didn't intend to lay spiritual overtones on the evening but couldn't help acknowledging that the whole thing felt like salvation, freedom in blistered feet, in sweat and rain and melting mascara. The night cracked wide open—raw, fleeting, beautiful, and rare.

I see that same wide open beauty in my clients. They are smart, engaging, sometimes fit, sometimes not-fit people who profoundly underestimate how extraordinary and capable they are. Their lives pulsate alternately with stagnation and transformation. They come to me for answers to a host of fitness conundrums and physical challenges, and I do my best to help them out. They look to me to be the expert, but I'm not really. I'm tossed and turned from clear and energized to lost and upended as often as any of them.

The only difference is that they are still at war with their bodies while I'm spinning off, out of the field of battle. They're good people with good intentions and bad habits. They're distracted and doing the best they can. They inch forward while I wait and watch for opportunities to nudge them along.

Every now and then one of them decides that it's time. They've had enough of things as they are. They pick up a heavy shovel, stick it in the ground, place one foot firmly on top and throw their entire weight into uprooting one little part of their lives in the hope that the upheaval will spread—unearthing the next, best version of themselves.

They stand in the dead heat of the blur in the bodies they have—and start moving. They grab hold of every hobby, passion, or person they can think of and keep going no matter what. There is no stopping. There might be plenty more bad days, but within those days they look for every opportunity they can find to reinforce their well-being.

And when they do that, it works, once and for all—and it makes me giddy just thinking about it. They stop running *away* from whatever it is that they hate and start running *toward* something they love.

A client who lost twenty-five pounds last year without dieting or deprivation told me recently, "I feel like I've dodged a bullet. I'm just overwhelmed that this is happening. I've been through a lot of healing emotionally in my life, and I know what it feels like to come out of that. But physically, I've been stuck in this rut. And I kept thinking, 'I don't feel like the emotional crap is still driving this.' I just felt like my body was a wreck, and I had poor eating habits as a result of all of those years. But I wanted my physical state to match where I was spiritually and emotionally.

"I started asking myself at every meal, 'What have I actually fed myself with, nourished myself with here?' I want to make sure there's something healthful in every meal and every snack. I don't eat after 7 o'clock most of the time, and I do protein in the morning. Big breakfast, medium lunch, light dinner. I realized I don't have to jump on every bandwagon. It's about paying attention to the subtle signs my body gives me. I've spent a lot of time reflecting and, honestly, grieving what I was doing to my body before. I was starving myself. I was eating all the time but starving my body of everything it could use."

Like so many of us, she was at war, and the rift with her body only got wider until she stopped going on the attack. She stopped dieting and stopped listening to anybody's voice other than her own about which food and exercise felt viscerally right. And after she stopped, she started making sure her body was fed with real, whole food and strengthening her muscles and bones with regular, pain-free bike rides and walks.

She switched her focus from restriction to healing.

When a client comes to me in search of a body she can barely imagine, the first thing I do, before tackling bad dietary habits or setting fitness goals, is to remind her what it feels like to breathe. Depending on her physical condition, I may do that on a treadmill, with a steady walk up a hill, or a series of sun salutations. Once we find breath, I go for strength: brute, physical strength. This is power. And once she feels powerful, she can decide what's next.

If she feels out of control with food, we come back to the breath. When she finds herself about to eat something she knows will ultimately make her feel awful, I ask her to hold her breath: breathe in; see the choice in front of her; see it; hold it; see it again; and exhale. From there, she can make the best decision she's capable of at the time, on to the next. If she toys with and bats this process around for a while, healthy choices will happen more often than not and become second nature over time.

If she shows up consistently in pursuit of getting better; gently and steadily pushes her boundaries; and commits to pressing on for as long as she has breath in her lungs, her body will get stronger and her life will reflect that change in ways she can't even conceive of beforehand. She will stop manipulating her body and start strengthening it.

She'll backslide now and then—everybody does—but with a growing reverence for what she's capable of and acceptance of where she's starting from, each day will present a fresh starting line, however fractured or flawless it might be.

There is a huge difference between acceptance and *giving up*. Acceptance is refuge, not resignation. It's a nonjudgmental recognition of the facts of your life and body. It allows you to see it all clearly enough that you can figure out what to *do* about it. It creates a situation where you are free to experiment with new routines, to see which new habit might challenge and move you along without creating a backlash.

Truth is power if you're not busy trying to deny it.

Fact: As of this writing, I am thirty-eight years old. I have a history of depression, food addiction, and messing up my body in all kinds of ways in the name of weight loss. I have been a student, an animal lover, a musician, a temp, a waitress, a human resources coordinator, a personal trainer, a writer, a wife, and most recently, a mom.

Also fact: The young woman with disordered eating habits, shattered by a fiancé who didn't want her, crippled by shame and embarrassment, and shackled to food for solace, lived fifteen years ago. She is long gone. She passed away with time and is sustained only by my memory.

I finally realized that there is no reason, other than my own choosing, that I *have* to have a screwed up relationship with food and my body going forward. There is no reason I have to continue to build my identity around being a chubby personal trainer with food and body issues. That story is not me, and I am not it. It served me well enough. It kept me going in a neutral, manageable sort of a way. It will always be part of who I am—and that's fine—but it doesn't own me. I realized that, if I want to, I always have the option of (1) letting it go and (2) trying something new.

Assuming our bodies and brains are functional—that we have sought whatever help we need from nutritionists, psychologists, and physicians—we all have the option to leave tired, old behaviors and habits of mind behind. But it can be as hard to let go as it is to forge ahead. Marinating in discomfort can seem easier than taking a risk, but staying willfully stuck is a tragic waste of time.

Life deals some incredibly difficult blows, but how we respond to those blows, both large and small, determines our experience. Beyond the obvious impact on relationships and state of mind, the choice between ruminating on past injustices or letting them fortify and inform us determines the state of our bodies, our blood pressure and heart rates, stress hormone levels, and very possibly how long and how well we will live.

The future is undetermined, but we forget how much power we possess simply by how we choose to respond. As Alice Walker wrote, "The most common way people give up their power is by thinking they don't have any."[1]

I take inspiration, on this front, from veterans, victims of tragedies such as terrorist attacks, and close friends and family who have suffered and are still suffering the ravages of cancer. They have wisdom to share about how to move forward, and those of us who do not suffer from such tragic circumstances would do well to listen.

An acquaintance of mine, blogger Joanna Montgomery, a forty-seven-year-old mom with terminal brain cancer wrote the following words seven weeks before her death: "I've had the benefit of time to clean out many of my closets; not just the literal ones in my home, but those stuffed with emotional baggage I've carried around far too long. I've known this intellectually all along, but I now know from experience that these resentments are not just unhealthy, but toxic, to both my physical and emotional body. I've learned that not using my voice—as both a mother and a human—only stifles my authentic self. . . . I can't help but marvel over how much time I've spent over the last several decades over-complicating the simplest of situations. I can't imagine ever going back to my old ways. I've seen behind the curtain. I'm awake. And I don't ever want to go back to sleep."[2]

Time's a-wasting. Wake up. Fulfillment and confidence have nothing to do with getting thin. They have everything to do with taking care of yourself and the people you love, speaking your mind, and contributing whatever you have to give to this crazy world we live in.

Defy the impulse to define yourself by your weight, and defy your friends when they try to do the same. You have the power in your own little universe to flip the conversation on its head—to instigate a new value system based on health, wisdom, contribution, and engagement. We're all in this together. Our individual struggles are very real, but they're not unique. We could all use a little lightening up.

Defining our worth based on body type is patently ridiculous.

There is no reason we have to lug around body baggage like it's our lot in life. Put it down. Walk away. Vocally, openly prioritize creativity and intelligence, and maybe, if we're steadfast in those values, the little kids coming up—the ones just now learning to utilize their own bodies, not old enough yet to have picked up their own baggage—might be able to enter adulthood lighter than we did, with more energy to spare for innovation and basic, unadulterated appreciation for their lives and bodies; for breathing, friendship, and love.

I used to believe that romantic love would be the thing that would set my body free. I thought a man could make me feel beautiful and validated, but as kind, insightful men, as well as cruel and thoughtless ones, came and went, I had to admit that no one (no matter how warm or loving) would ever possess the special skills to make me feel okay in my skin. I had to do that on my own, and that shift had everything to do with what I chose to value.

Peace ended up coming in the form of appreciation for a hot shower; a warm bed to crawl into; a cat sleeping on my head; a puppy sleeping at my feet; a friend to make me laugh until I cried; a mountain that stood ready to be climbed; and a concert that left me staring at the stars. Creature comforts and dear friends.

If you measure success and worthiness based on anybody else's approval or a particular number on the scale, you will never be free. The sun cannot rise and fall with your weight. It's variable, and you are human. Your body is a vehicle for being, something worth caring for that is yours and yours alone. If it feels like it's on the right track, you have due cause for celebration. And if you feel yourself clamping down or tensing up, grasping for control and getting ready to fight, turn without a second thought, back to the habits and people that you know for a fact will keep you afloat.

Without the catalyst of a crisis, it's undeniably difficult to break out of well-worn neurological ruts, but it is absolutely possible. Just do something new; try something. Keep experimenting, and be purposeful. Fancy yourself both a visionary and a worker bee. Do what you can—a little something new every day.

In New York City, before I had any idea what I was doing or why, I wandered through Central Park on weekends or walked fifty or sixty blocks home from work at night because it felt like a good thing to do. I wasn't trying to lose weight. I knew I was stress eating way too much for that to happen. I walked because it cleared my head. I had a choice between doing something good or not, and thought, rather than being a wreck all the time, it might be a good idea to try to do something good whenever possible. So I wandered the streets, breathing in sunshine and air, and every time, they brought me back to life.

Years later in California, with no job or money, I set out on daily hikes in search of that same life-giving sunshine and air. No matter how broke or busy I was, no matter what landscape I was facing, I found relief in hiking and breathing and enough clarity to make better, more nourishing decisions.

I finally woke up one day, followed by a week and then a year, without feeling like food had more power than I did, so I kept at it, kept right on walking en route to a life that felt steadily better. I had no idea where I was headed half the time but kept on, fully prepared for a lifetime of steady steps. I was bullheaded about it, unwilling to live with the alternative, doing whatever I could, however small it might be, to move toward better and away from worse: daily walks; nutrition classes; cities explored; books read; new friends; reliable and not-so-reliable jobs; workouts before work; lunches in Tupperware; broken bones; a few bad break-ups; a cheap guitar; and far too many words on paper.

And when I found myself under streetlights with arms outstretched in a body that felt like heaven on earth, I couldn't believe how young I was. I was caught off guard by the fact that it didn't take a lifetime. I wasn't an old lady yet. I had many more decades to go, and all I had to do to maintain that brilliant state of being was to nourish myself rather than beating myself down—and reinvest every ounce of attention and love I could muster back into my clients and friends after they had given me so much by letting me bear witness to the frustration and transformation of their lives and bodies.

In her TED talk, "The Danger of a Single Story," Chimamanda Ngozi Adichie said, "When we reject the single story, when we realize that there is never a single story . . . we regain a kind of paradise."[3] Freedom.

Standing where I am now, mostly unburdened, having witnessed so many single stories splinter and spread wide open, I have learned the following:

1. Start where you are.
2. Do something good that feels good *now*, not something that supposedly will make you feel good later. If jogging around the block feels like a nightmare, don't do it. Don't do *anything* that even vaguely resembles a nightmare. Skip it, and figure out what turns you on. This is the incredibly beautiful dance between indulgence and strength, between Lothario and the Cheerleader. Find healthy indulgences that bring you to life, and revisit them relentlessly.
3. Eat for your body, and exercise for your mind. Food can lighten you, and exercise can lift your spirits. *Feed* your body with both fuel and motion. Utilize it.
4. Show up for yourself like you do for your child, mother, or best friend. Show up; shut up; pay attention—and do whatever you can to make it all better.
5. Allow changes to take root. Let assumptions about who you are and what you're capable of morph over time.

That last point is a squirrelly one. Success is notoriously slippery. It feels unstable, simultaneously exciting and fickle. It's foreign, and as long as something is foreign, it's about as secure as an armload full of golf balls. The tighter you grip, the harder it is to hold on.

When you start to achieve goals that were previously just fantasies, there's a tendency to feel like you might be about to face-plant. Things seem a little too good, a little too smooth, like it's been a little too long since everything fell apart.

In her book, *Daring Greatly*, Brene Brown has a name for this phenomenon: "foreboding joy."[4] Progress can be terrifying if you're afraid it's about to slip away—but if you allow that fear to send you back into battle against your body, you are almost guaranteed to lose whatever headway you've made. If you clamp down, you will backslide.

The only thing to do in the face of that fear is *reengage* with whatever got you there in the first place. Lean on your fallback habits. Lean on the things that strengthen you. That's what they're there for. It's one system, the same system all the time, no matter the circumstances.

If you stick with it, you'll find yourself running into the final challenge, the biggest one, the one that indicates that you have finally, officially arrived at a new version of yourself.

A few weeks or months after you've hit a major goal, the ground will shift underneath you. You'll feel puffy again. Your clothes will seem tighter than they did the day before, but the scale will show that you're holding steady. You'll be capable of running farther and faster than ever before, but will suddenly feel weighed down again. The elation you had when you first hit your goal will bounce away, just out of reach.

Your new, transformed body will begin feeling *normal*, like your regular old self, and that normalcy will erase the sensation of breaking through that you were feeding on to keep the good juju coming.

This is a signal that your body is aching for the next step—because there is always a next step to getting healthier and stronger. It does not mean that you have failed or that you're about to fail. It's a sign that you've accomplished what you set out to do. Your body has settled in;

your brain has caught up; and you feel just like you did before, lumpy in the same old spots.

If this happens to you, call up your soul shine people and cry tears of joy because this is the ultimate victory. You have arrived at the culmination of your hard work. You set out to create a different definition of normal—at a lighter weight in a stronger body, without the struggle—and here it is. But with that accomplishment, you're still you. Your body still has the same oddities, and your heart still breaks in the same ways. Lothario lurks, and old impulses rise up in stressful times.

In this moment, you are precariously susceptible to the forces that trounced you in the first place, but if you understand what is happening, and know to turn away from those forces rather than engaging in a fight, you can come back again to your infrastructure, resilient and indestructible.

Fill your life with things that feed and fulfill you, and let a new personal story emerge of someone powerful, dynamic, and generous. Stay open to the possibility that you can appreciate your body for what it is, while simultaneously molding the best version of it that you possibly can. We're at our best when we take care.

For me, that sometimes means dark chocolate, sometimes means a pedicure when I probably shouldn't be spending the money, and sometimes means drinking a little too much and dancing myself to distraction with girlfriends in a dark nightclub. Most of the time, though, taking care of myself means dragging my butt out of bed, putting on my sneakers, and taking a few steps down the street—which leads to ten minutes and then twenty and then thirty, a vigorous heart rate, open lungs, a rush of adrenaline, and knowing for the rest of the day that I feel better than I did before because I pried myself loose. I don't need to be someone with six-pack abs. All I need to be is agile, energized, and full of breath.

I went jogging at a park near my house recently that has a small lake at the center of it. As I stood aimlessly staring at the water, an old man strolled by with a fishing pole propped up on his shoulder. "You ain't gone but a mile," he said with a wink.

Yes, sir, too true—but I have pet all the puppies; I have watched the cranes lift off and land; jotted down an idea; talked to my best friend; and looked up at the sky. I'd say that mile was well-lived.

He found a perch lakeside and settled in to begin his day, while I turned my attention to my playlist. I cranked up the volume, and dug in, up a long, hilly, twisting road, half-running/half-hiking, sweating from every pore, hot as blazes. I was wide open, heading home to my three-year-old little man and his precious pit bull.

In a past lifetime, I would have felt like I had been busted, like I was breaking the cardinal rule of wellness, "No pain, no gain." I would have accused myself of all sorts of nasty things: laziness and being a fat ass among them. But not anymore. If my time is well spent, if my body is awake and alive, there is no need for a preconceived notion of what constitutes an effective workout.

If I'm paying attention, I can sense how much or how little my body needs on any given day to feel challenged and supported; and, thankfully, over time I have learned to read my clients' bodies as well, to determine whether they need to pound out aggression, to stretch and breathe, or somewhere in between.

They will unravel their own food-loving, body-bashing, triumphant, and conflicted stories in time. All I can do is encourage them to find strength from the outside in; one weight, one mile, one freefall at a time.

And my own story—without question—will always include eating more Mexican food than I need on a Sunday afternoon with Sophia in the old neighborhood, and putting on my sneakers when I don't feel like it. I will occasionally be found barefoot in the dust at a music festival or wandering through a farmer's market, trying to figure out what the hell a parsnip is. And I'll probably always have an ache inside for the simple silence of a red velvet cupcake—and that's just fine with me.

There is no way my seventy-year-old lady will have time for books like this—too many dogs to play with, too many hikes to take. By then, I plan to be long gone, long since done with this conversation. By then, I plan on having, in the wise words of songwriter Abe Wilson, "one less thing to give a damn about."[5]

For the next thirty-five years or so, you'll find me on a long walk from here to the cliffs over Malibu. I look forward to the clients I'll meet on the way. They'll teach me and join me for a bit, before turning off in search of their own weathered, old ladies—arm-in-arm with Lothario and the Cheerleader—with numerous pit stops along the way for cocktails and a taste of local flavor. Hopefully, in time, they will feel their way through the days and nights until they find themselves wandering all alone on a summer evening with arms outstretched under streetlights. Liberated, at whatever weight works.

Beauty, cracked wide open.

TOOLBOX

Four things:

1. Recognize when you feel out of control and weighed down.
2. Do something physically different. Uproot. Pry yourself loose.
3. Walk directly through whatever doors open. Explore relentlessly.
4. When you start to slip, come back to your core habits. Rest, regroup, and start again.

AFTERWORD

Don't Go It Alone

So here you are at the end of the book, awash in bright and shiny words, a whole lot of "whoop-whoop!" and "do what you love!" But as we all know, rather than sticking with some of the changes you just made, what you're most likely to do at this point is put the book down until the next time you get inspired or frustrated. By then you'll be back where you started, and the cycle will continue as usual. If you don't want that to happen, if, instead, you want to see real changes, you need one more thing.

You need somebody—preferably several somebodies—to call you out on an ongoing basis. You need a group of people who hold no sway over you at work or at home to hold you accountable, some folks to help you keep it together.

Before I dive any deeper on this, I have to confess that I hate groups. I do very badly when it comes to joining things and sticking with them. I prefer to be aimless. I despise rules and schedules and am generally averse to any kind of institutional situation. But here's the thing: We need other human beings to look us in the face on a regular basis and ask us how it's going. That fact is unfortunate for introverts like myself, but it's true. I know this because—after years of studying and practicing this stuff, working out and training clients—I didn't get anywhere near where I wanted to go until I put together a band of like-minded misfits for support and accountability. It didn't matter what I did for a living. I still needed outside reinforcement when I found myself clinging precariously to the edge of a good day. I needed my tribe.

Maybe you're the anomaly, the one who can pull it off by yourself, but for most of us, it doesn't work to do it alone. Life is too distracting. Without somebody else to hold up a mirror, we're lost. It's too easy to lose perspective and fall back into old patterns without even realizing it.

If you don't want to spend the rest of your life in a perpetual sling-shot, bouncing back and forth, losing consciousness and coming to your senses with bad habits (and your weight) spiking out of control, you need a grounding force to keep you focused.

The good news is that you don't have to sign up for this forced accountability with anybody else's people. You can do it with *your* people in your house, with your beverages and vibe. You can do it in your tiny, little apartment or on your palatial estate. You can sit on the floor or around a kitchen table. You can even do it online via video conference call if your people are far away, just make sure you can see each other's faces.

You're the boss of how it goes down, but the bottom line is that you and whoever you enlist can help each other out by simply showing up, shooting the shit, and bearing witness to each other's lives with a steady eye on getting healthier.

So here's how to start your own group.

(I'll pause here for laughter.)

Yes, I'm talking about putting together a group—an irreverent, unconventional wellness group made up of people who, like you, want to prioritize health but maybe can't afford to (or don't want to) see a personal trainer or a shrink. Call it what you will: your tribe, your lightness group, your strength club, your merry band of mindful misfits. My original group goes by Tribe because we feel innately invested in each other's well-being and blissfully out of step with the fitness and weight loss culture at large. We are a world apart, dedicated to wellness in our own subversive, quirky, little ways. (Plus, there is a gay bar in Nashville called Tribe with the best boys, drinks, and tunes in town, and we take serious inspiration from the good times happening over there.)

Everybody knows that too many hours on the couch and eating too much for the wrong reasons will make you feel worse. And we all know that getting some exercise or eating something real makes you better. Nobody in the group has to be a personal trainer to know that. The task at hand is for you and your fellow misfits to regularly remind each other to keep moving toward better by inserting as many healthy habits as you comfortably can into your days—and when you find yourself most definitely *not* moving toward better, *keep showing up anyway*. Press on in whatever way you can.

Steady accountability demands action. People in the group inevitably become witnesses to what is and isn't working. If you're stuck in the same rut for long enough—talking about the same issue over and over again to neutral observers—you're eventually going to hone in on what needs changing. Once it's obvious to everyone in the room, including you, what is not working, they can help you brainstorm about what to do next. They can help you pimp out your cage.

The most incredible, enlightening thing happens when you find yourself actively listening to smart, beautiful people of all sizes, who are judging and limiting themselves based on physical flaws that either don't exist or don't matter to anyone but them. The whole thing starts to look nuts.

You look and listen and realize that we're all repeating the same mantras and trying to fit into the same meaningless, narrow ideals. You can see perfectly clearly that those lovely people are all totally fine and worthy of every good thing in life—and you realize like a lightning bolt to the brain that you might be fine too.

You begin to see how much easier it is for them to make productive decisions when they put their focus on *doing* something rather than *not* doing something—and, with that recognition, you find your way to a few new, clear, unemotional, healthy decisions of your own.

As a group, instead of trying to get *skinny*, you decide to collectively become the best, easiest, strongest, most lighthearted versions of your-selves possible, with all of the accompanying bulges and bumps, a feel-ing a friend of mine once referred to as "miracle easy."

The idea is to get three to ten people in a room every two weeks who want to spout off about whatever is happening and raise a glass to good health, with an eye on making their bodies and lives stronger and more vibrant in the process.

In theory, you can do this with just one other person, but I've found that it's best to have at least two. You need more than one because if your one and only person gets distracted or discouraged (which they will at some point because we're all human), they will leave you in the lurch and, from there, all of the forward motion will be left up to you, which is no different than doing it alone, maybe even harder because you've just been abandoned.

Everyone of every size is welcome—and I'm not just talking about the big girls. (In fact, I'm not just talking about women. You can invite boys to come along too.) My original group has had members ranging from one hundred to four hundred pounds. Everyone has different issues, and everyone's concerns are valid. We are all in a different spot, but we're all heading in the same direction.

When I sent out the first email asking my friends and acquaintances if they wanted to do this with me, I was embarrassed to admit that I still had food and body issues and felt presumptuous assuming that they might have the same. Worse, I knew I would have to start from a place of truth. I wanted to project an image of having it all together, to be the fearless leader, but I understood that the only way to lead would be to lay my frustration and confusion out for all to see, just like I was asking them to do—and allow them to help me as much as I would be helping them. It's one thing to be authentic with words on paper and another to speak truth to the faces of the women I know and love from my actual life.

I hit send, held my breath, and waited. To my dismay, the response was swift and enthusiastic. Eight women jumped aboard, and I had no choice but to follow through.

The people who showed up for that first meeting—and have continued to show up for over three years—have created a paradigm shift in their minds. They have switched their focus from weight to well-being, and the results have been remarkable.

We joke that the group should have a disclaimer: Be warned that if you join this group you will probably end up changing jobs, breaking up with a lover, falling in love, having a baby, moving, going back to school, or running a marathon. It's amazing how difficult it becomes to stay stuck when you have a gaggle of people prodding and cheering you on.

When we first started, most of them didn't know each other. I was the common denominator, but over time, they have come to rely on each other. Everybody approaches the process in her own way, but the overall objective for every one of us is to keep moving forward. We set small goals, always focused on what can be *added* to our lives rather than taken away, and check in two weeks later to see if we pulled it off.

Sometimes people show up in a state of upheaval. We listen if they want to talk, or hand them a tissue and move on if they don't. Meetings usually last about an hour to an hour and a half. Most of the time we're laughing by the end about how weird and awkward it is to split an entrée with your judgmental mom at a restaurant; or how infuriatingly idiotic the jerk in the corner office is when he calls you "sweetheart" on your way to lunch every day.

Some people are training for 10Ks, while others are just trying to stand up at their desks for five minutes. A lot of them are dealing with sick kids, aging parents, or jobs they deeply dislike. There are money and fertility issues, injuries and car accidents. There are engagements and promotions, graduations and newborns. There's no singular experience, and there are certainly no uniform expectations. We are all perpetually triumphant and falling apart in our own unique ways, and it's all to be expected.

They have kept my head above water when I wanted to stop treading and slip into the deep, and if any of them ever called in the middle of the night, I would get out of bed and pick them up by the side of the road—no questions asked. A wink maybe, but no questions asked. They are my people.

I confess that making time for the meetings can be a minor hassle; it's certainly more of a hassle than sitting on my butt and watching a movie. I straighten up my house every other Monday night for these people. I clear my schedule and get a sitter for my kid if my husband isn't around. I have to make sure there are enough clean glasses and generally expect one or two people who say they're coming to flake last minute because that's just how it goes.

It can be a hassle for me, and they openly admit that it's not easy for them at times either. They get home from work and are tired. They want to pack it in for the night but have to get up and out again. They can't put on their PJ pants just yet, unless that's how they want to roll in. Like any other helpful, new habit, it's hard to remember how good it feels to show up when you're oh-so-tempted by the couch. But they do show up, and I open the door. And we never regret it. We are always reminded in the end to support and strengthen our bodies, and we're always shocked at how quickly and easily we forget to do just that in the course of our regular lives.

It costs us a little something. We put in our time and show up every two weeks. It takes a bit of effort, but when you start to see the people around you expanding—stretching their potential, thinking outside of the box, and doing things you never thought they would free themselves to do—you can't help but get inspired.

Human beings mirror the behavior and activities of the people around them. We gain momentum from each other. Goodness spreads—and so does courage, and so does weight loss.

Forming a "Tribe" of your own really isn't all that difficult, and it could be the key, finally, to a much improved life and body. All you need is an email invitation and some wine. Or coffee. Or whatever your poison.

If you want to start your own group, do it your way. But whatever you do, make sure there are no judgments—whether someone is struggling with not eating enough, eating too much, or finding the motivation to step out the front door—there should be no back-stabbing or competition. People may come for a few months, disappear for a while and come back again, and that's fine too. Meet everybody right where they are.

Redefine "lightness" for yourselves. Take back as many minutes of your lives as you can, *as soon as you can*. Pound into your collective consciousness that freedom (and, yes, weight loss) come from the pursuit of pleasure, not pain. Speak out loud whatever it is that's happening; take its breath away. And give yourself permission to change over time to move; to quit; to eat a piece of fruit; to initiate a new friendship; to take up a new hobby; to ask for a raise; to declutter; or to stand up and walk out. Do *your* thing, whatever that might be, unapologetically.

I am a trainer who hates to run. That seems strange to most people, but it makes my body hurt in a not-good way; and I have to honor that. What I usually need more than anything is a walk, a yoga class, some free weights, and bath salts, but occasionally an urge arises out of nowhere to launch into a sprint—chest out, arms pumping—and I have to honor that too. Like anything else, it comes in waves.

So sprint when you can and walk when you can, and love it all in equal measure. Go looking for what turns you on, be it dirty dancing or bird watching. But whatever you do, don't stop looking; don't stop stretching; and don't let your people stop either.

When we exercise a muscle, it burns because (by stressing it) we are intentionally creating tiny tears in the muscle fibers. When the tears heal, the fibers get sturdier. It's called muscle hypertrophy, and it's the mechanism by which we get stronger, a process of pushing beyond what's comfortable and allowing time to heal.

You have to rip your life open a little before it can grow, but alone in a room, it can be difficult to see when it's been too long since you stretched beyond your bounds. You need someone there to notice and mark the passage of time. Measured bouts of conscious stretching, tiny tears, can make you stronger if you let them. The gathering is a place to test and push your boundaries. It creates structured accountability for steady advancement with built-in reinforcements.

The upside for you as the founder of the group is that all eyes are on you to keep growing into and through the freefall. You might fall apart for a minute, but you'll get up again and keep going because you'll want to set an example, to keep the whole operation from getting stuck in the mud. You'll climb up and out of your ditch, gladiator-style, and keep stumbling forward, out of the field of battle and into fields of daisies (yep, daisies)—leading the charge toward better and away from worse.

Life is incredibly, profoundly fragile. Don't waste it worrying about cellulite. Eat a cupcake and go hiking instead—and take your people with you.

The following are a few suggestions to help you form your group. If you have questions, success stories, or struggles to share, tweet me @strengthoutside, or visit www.strengthoutsidein.com for additional resources.

To start your own Tribe:

1. Find your people—send out an email or put up a notice on social media, at your school, workplace, or church. You're looking for people who want to actively pursue better health in a gentle but purposeful way. The group is about body acceptance, but it's also about forward motion and steady improvement. The meetings are a place to acknowledge difficulties, not to get bogged down in them.

2. Arrange a time and place to meet—I recommend once every two weeks. Once a month allows too much time to go by before being accountable to the group again, and weekly meetings can place too high a demand on people's time, which makes it difficult to commit long

term. Make sure you have a comfortable place to sit where you can see each other. Personally, I think everything is always better when pets are present for slobbering and snoozing, but that might be unique to my brand of bleeding heart, animal-loving folks. Again, your group is your own. Make it comfy, whatever that means for you.

3. The group is and always should be free, but at each of our meetings in Nashville, we put a bowl off to the side to accept donations for our local food bank on a voluntary basis. No one is watching who does or doesn't give. It's *completely* optional. It's up to you whether or not to accept donations at your meetings, but if you do, my only request is that the money raised go to a food or clean water-related charity. Let's nurture other people's bodies while we nurture our own.

4. To make your meeting both functional and relaxed, you'll need a notebook and something to drink. Put someone in charge of writing down everybody's goals in a single notebook or online forum and bringing that information to each meeting. People have a tendency to rewrite their goals in their minds, often convincing themselves that they have failed when they actually succeeded. I keep the notebook for our group since we meet at my house.

If you want drinks, assign that responsibility to a different person each meeting, or you, as the host, can provide whatever you want. How you split up those responsibilities is up to you. If you have a champion boozer who wants to be in charge of drinks all the time, go for it. Note: The boozer and the person in charge of goalkeeping should probably not be the same person.

5. At the first meeting and/or anytime somebody new comes, explain the two core principles of the group: (1) The central idea is to move toward better and away from worse. (2) We do that by adding good things to crowd out the bad, through exploration, not deprivation.

6. Once everyone is settled in, go around the room. Anyone who wants to contribute can say what challenges they are facing with their health; what aspects of their life might be getting in the way; what habits they would like to change; what their experience has been while trying to meet their goals since the last meeting; and any other con-

cerns. You'll find all kinds of issues coming up (for example, stress, insomnia, work, family, snacking, PMS). Allow space for open discussion. It doesn't need to be an "I speak, then you speak, then the next person speaks" kind of a situation. As I said, shoot the shit. It should be relaxed, but make sure everybody gets a chance. This first part of the discussion isn't about setting new goals or projecting into upcoming weeks. It's just about taking a look at what is currently happening and looking for patterns and obstacles. Save goals for the second time around the room, and anyone who doesn't want to speak shouldn't feel pressured.

7. Move on to goals. Each person should set a goal to fulfill over the following two weeks. They can range from "coming back to this meeting next time" to "eating one piece of fruit per day"; from "drinking three bottles of water at work each day" to "going to the gym twice a week." Some people like to set one nutrition and one fitness goal, which is fine, but they should be easily attainable. If a goal seems too lofty, the group should encourage the person to scale it back. Long-term goals are valid and important, but short-term behavior changes are the centerpiece of the group and the engine that powers long-term change. Go around the circle, and allow each person to set a goal or two for the following meeting. They should be individual and small. Make it something you're pretty damn sure you can walk in the door two weeks later and say, "I did it!"

For instance, a woman who watches TV while eating breakfast and dinner every day decides that she wants to set a goal not to eat in front of the TV at all. Encourage her to shoot for breakfast first. Or dinner on Mondays and Tuesdays. If her goals are too abrupt or too big, she'll probably fail. It's best to make them smaller at first. If the change turns out to be easy, she can push it further at the next meeting and set a bigger goal.

Use the group to challenge whether each goal seems attainable. If someone can articulate why a larger goal isn't a failure waiting to happen, allow that and be prepared to either join in the celebration or pick up the pieces. Sometimes people thrive on lofty fitness goals, especially if they are already athletes.

8. From the updates and goals, the conversation will wander. Let it. Unexpected insights, recipes, books, and ideas will emerge. Tangents lead to interesting places.

9. Keep up with each other between meetings. Set up a private group page online where members can post if anything comes to mind. Say, for example, you're sitting in your car in the parking lot of the gym, trying to convince yourself to go inside, instead of reclining and taking a nap in your bucket seat. Post it. Or the woman who is trying not to watch TV during breakfast or dinner can post updates. Maybe you found a great app to track your morning bike ride or organize meal planning. It's a place to reach out for reinforcements or share a cool quote or some good vibes if you have them to spare.

10. Keep meeting. Let people quit who want to quit, and welcome newcomers. Let people fail. If they don't meet their goals, that's fine. It's part of the process. At least they showed up. If a goal isn't met, scale it back or try a different one. Keep moving in the right general direc-tion, and if somebody has a big win—ten pounds lost or a shit ex-boyfriend dumped—celebrate and celebrate big. When one person takes a big step forward, everybody benefits.

We popped a champagne bottle in my group for the last three meet-ings in a row. One person quit her job, another got engaged, and an-other had a baby.

The tribe is, at its root, an external reinforcement of mindfulness. It's a structural practice of observing what isn't working and implement-ing new things that will work better. It's relaxed and informal, basically just an excuse to get together with friends a couple of times a month. There will be tears, but you'll be surprised how often they will be tears of relief. It's exciting when people realize that they don't have to beat themselves up in order to get better, but it's also emotional. The first time they lose weight or find themselves standing taller by taking care of themselves instead of dieting, they tend to be both thrilled and heartbroken—thrilled by the accomplishment and heartbroken by how much time and energy they wasted going at it bass-ackward.

I suppose there are women in the world who walk around judging each other's bodies and minds, but based on my people, I don't know who they are. And I don't care to. Body baggage is something we all carry with us to one degree or another, but it's also something we can leave behind. Our best bet for doing that—our best chance to shift our values, stick with the process, build healthier bodies, and pass it all down—is to do it together.

Find people you enjoy; gather them in your home or church basement or around your backyard fire pit; and hold on for dear life when somebody loses a loved one, a rejection letter arrives, or the cold, long, chill of winter slithers its way under your skin. Be each other's life force, and keep each other from slipping too far, for too long. If somebody does slip, keep vigil at the edge of the ditch until they are ready to reach up, climb out, and sit down again, present and accounted for. Together, you will find your footing, and if you keep showing up, you *will* get better. Lighter.

ACKNOWLEDGMENTS

I could not have completed this book if it weren't for the tireless encouragement, insight, diatribes, non-sequiturs, and air drumming of my best friend and lover, Ken. Thanks for walking on the outside.

J, you have read every draft of every phase of this book with a keen eye on storytelling. It would be a muddled monstrosity without you. Thanks for being my person. Here's to every bit of mayhem, past and future.

T, our backyard, moonlit ruminations provided countless sparks of inspiration and uprooted my brain when I needed it the most. You are wise beyond your years. Now go put some clothes on. You're scaring the neighbors.

Suzanne Staszak-Silva, though I generally had to step away from my computer to reinforce my sanity with one of my core healthy habits after receiving your notes, I have to concede that your guidance and persistent focus on making these stories accessible made this book infinitely better. Thank you for being a hard ass. There, I said it. And thanks to the rest of the team at Rowman and Littlefield—Elaine, Jackie, Kathryn, and Crystal—who kept me in the loop and answered all of my nine million questions.

Allison Cohen, you have officially been dubbed "the unicorn" around here. Get used to it.

Friends, clients, and members of the original Tribe: Katrina, JJ, Emily 1, Emily 2, Karen, Annie, Lindsay, Lauren, Linnet, Angela, Jennifer, Sumeeta, Ana Lee, Sally, Nikki, Wendy, Traci, Julia, Ali, Katie, Kate, Claire, Jessica, Christine, Glen, Seth, and Steve—you have kept me sane and taught me everything I know about how to live stronger. Thank you for trusting me with your bodies and stories.

Mom, your devotion to wellness in underserved populations has had a far greater impact on me than you will ever know. Dad, thanks for making peacefulness matter and for teaching me that Dunkin' Donuts is a perfectly reasonable remedy for writer's block at midnight. We may not always use the same language, but I'm pretty sure we're talking about the same thing.

And to Sky, my baby boy, I never knew a little man could be so kind and so wise. By peeking out at the world in the way you do, you have shown me that everything is better when it's upside-down, that time is precious, and that a healthy body and curious mind are truly the greatest gifts any of us could ever hope to have.

NOTES

3. DAY AND NIGHT

1. This is paraphrased from memory, but its essence is intact. Archivists at the Ram Dass Organization were unable to put their hands on the lecture without more specific information about the date and location it was recorded, but they were familiar with the story and verified its existence.

2. National Suicide Prevention Hotline: 800-273-8255; National Eating Disorders Hotline: 800-931-2237; Crisis Call Center: 800-273-8255.

3. Thistle Farms: http://www.thistlefarms.org.

4. DIG THE RIDE

1. See Mignon's smile come alive on video at http://www.cupcakecollection.com/press.

2. Neale Donald Walsch, http://www.nealedonaldwalsch.com/.

3. James Hamblin, "Wine and Exercise: A Promising Combination," *The Atlantic*, September 3, 2014, http://www.theatlantic.com/health/archive/2014/09/working-with-the-wine-not-against-it/379504/.

5. HELP YOUR BRAIN HELP YOU

1. Cited from 2015 interview with Dr. Julie Price, PsyD, licensed clinical health psychologist, Vanderbilt University.

2. Sharon Begley, *Train Your Mind, Change Your Brain: How a New Science Reveals Our Extraordinary Potential to Transform Ourselves* (New York: Ballantine Books, 2007).

3. Charles Duhigg, *The Power of Habit: Why We Do What We Do in Life and Business* (New York: Random House, 2012), 283.

7. DODGING THE YO-YO

1. Michelle May, "Experts Speak Out about the Harmful Effects of Dieting," *Huffington Post*, http://www.huffingtonpost.com/michelle-may-md/yoyo-dieting_b_1887283.html.

2. Kenrya Rankin, "End the Yo-Yo Diet Cycle," *Fitness Magazine*, http://www.fitnessmagazine.com/weight-loss/tips/end-the-yo-yo-diet-cycle/; Kathleen Zelman, "Things You Should Never Do to Lose Weight." WebMD, 2011, http://www.webmd.com/diet/obesity/lose-weight-dangers.

9. DO SOMETHING

1. Arlene Weintraub, "Make Over Your Metabolism-Really!" *MORE Magazine*, April 2014, http://www.more.com/health/wellness/four-ways-to-make-over-your-metabolism.

2. Mandy Oaklander, "What Diet Soda Does to Belly Fat," *Time*, May 17, 2015, http://time.com/3746047/diet-soda-bad-belly-fat/; Julia Merz, "This Is How Diet Soda Can Make You Gain Weight," *Prevention*, September 22, 2014, http://www.prevention.com/health/diabetes/artificial-sweeteners-diet-soda-affect-gut-bacteria-and-weight-gain.

3. "Monterey Bay Aquarium Seafood Watch," http://www.montereybayaquarium.org/cr/cr_seafoodwatch/sfw_recommendations.aspx.

4. Hilary Parker, "A Sweet Problem: Princeton Researchers Find That High-Fructose Corn Syrup Prompts Considerably More Weight Gain," Princeton University, March 22, 2010, http://www.princeton.edu/main/news/archive/S26/91/22K07/index.xml?section=topstories.

5. "High Cholesterol. Trans Fat: Avoid This Cholesterol Double Whammy," June 19, 2015, http://www.mayoclinic.org/diseases-conditions/high-blood-cholesterol/in-depth/trans-fat/art-20046114.

6. Michael J. Breus, "Can't Lose Weight? Get Some Sleep," WebMD, http://www.webmd.com/diet/obesity/cant-shed-those-pounds.

10. MINDFULNESS AND MINDLESSNESS

1. Maurice Sendak, *Where the Wild Things Are* (New York: Harper & Row, 1963).

2. Pema Chödrön, *When Things Fall Apart: Heart Advice for Difficult Times* (Boston, MA: Shambhala, 1997).

3. Nicole Avena, Pedro Rada, and Bartley Hoebel, "Evidence for Sugar Addiction: Behavioral and Neurochemical Effects of Intermittent, Excessive Sugar Intake," *Neuroscience and Biobehavioral Reviews*, May 18, 2007.

4. Johann Hari, *Chasing the Scream: The First and Last Days of the War on Drugs* (New York: Bloomsbury USA, 2015).

5. http://www.huffingtonpost.com/johann-hari/the-real-cause-of-addic-ti_b_6506936.html

6. "14 Shocking Heroin Relapse Statistics—HRF," *HRF*, August 26, 2014, http://healthresearchfunding.org/shocking-heroin-relapse-statistics/.

7. "Find the Best Drug or Alcohol Addiction Recovery Helplines," Drug and Alcohol Recovery Hotlines—Toll-Free Substance Abuse Treatment Advisors, 888-966-8334. http://www.recovery.org/.

11. STARTING WHERE YOU ARE

1. S. J. Kentish, T. A. O'Donnell, C. L. Frisby, H. Li, G. A. Wittert, A. J. Page, "Altered Gastric Vagal Mechanosensitivity in Diet-Induced Obesity Persists on Return to Normal Chow and Is Accompanied by Increased Food Intake," *International Journal of Obesity*, 2013; DOI:10.1038/ijo.2013.138.

2. "Tree Change Dolls," Tree Change Dolls®, http://treechange-dolls.tumblr.com/; "IAmElemental Action Figures for Girls." http://www.iamelemental.com/.

12. WIDE OPEN

1. Alice Walker, "The Official Website for the American Novelist Poet," http://alicewalkersgarden.com/.

2. Joanna Montgomery, "Alive and Kicking," June 6, 2015, http://hellojo-mo.com/blog/alive-and-kicking/.

3. Chimamanda Ngozi Adichie, "The Danger of a Single Story," July 2009, http://www.ted.com/talks/chimaman-da_adichie_the_danger_of_a_single_story?language=en.

4. Brene Brown, *Daring Greatly: How the Courage to Be Vulnerable Transforms the Way We Live, Love, Parent, and Lead* (New York: Gotham Books, 2012).

5. Abe Wilson, "Light a Light," Sons of Bill. *Love and Logic*, 2014.

SELECTED BIBLIOGRAPHY

Begley, Sharon. *Train Your Mind, Change Your Brain: How a New Science Reveals Our Extraordinary Potential to Transform Ourselves*. New York: Ballantine Books, 2007.

Brown, Brene. *Daring Greatly: How the Courage to Be Vulnerable Transforms the Way We Live, Love, Parent, and Lead*. New York: Gotham Books, 2012.

Chödrön, Pema. *When Things Fall Apart: Heart Advice for Difficult Times*. Boston, MA: Shambhala, 1997.

Dillard, Annie. *The Writing Life*. New York: Harper & Row, 1989.

Duhigg, Charles. *The Power of Habit: Why We Do What We Do in Life and Business*. New York: Random House, 2012.

Hari, Johann. *Chasing the Scream: The First and Last Days of the War on Drugs*. New York: Bloomsbury USA, 2015.

Sendak, Maurice. *Where the Wild Things Are*. New York: Harper & Row, 1963.

Wilson, Abe. "Brand New Paradigm." Sons of Bill, *Love and Logic*, 2014.

FURTHER READINGS

The Blue Zones: Lessons for Living Longer from the People Who've Lived the Longest, by Dan Buettner. National Geographic, 2010.

Born Round: The Secret History of a Full-Time Eater, by Frank Bruni. Penguin Books, 2010.

Broken Open: How Difficult Times Can Help Us Grow, by Elizabeth Lesser. Villard Books, 2005.

The China Study: Startling Implications for Diet, Weight Loss and Long-Term Health, by T. Colin Campbell, PhD, and Thomas M. Campbell II, MD. BenBella Books, 2006.

Drive: The Surprising Truth about What Drives Us, by Daniel Pink. Riverhead Books, 2011.

The End of Overeating: Taking Control of the Insatiable American Appetite, by David A. Kessler. Rodale Books, 2010.

In Defense of Food: An Eater's Manifesto, by Michael Pollan. Penguin, 2009.

Kitchen Yoga: Simple Home Practices to Transform Mind, Body, and Life, by Melanie Salvatore-August. Yellow Pear Press, 2015.

No Sweat: How the Simple Science of Motivation Can Bring You a Lifetime of Fitness, by Michelle Segar, PhD. AMACOM, 2015.

Traveling Mercies: Some Thoughts on Faith, by Anne Lamott. Anchor, 2000.

Truth and Beauty: A Friendship, by Ann Patchett. Harper Perennial, 2005.

Your Body Is Awesome: Body Respect for Children, by Sigrun Danielsdottier and Bjork Bjarkadottir (illustrator). Singing Dragon, 2014.

Wild: From Lost to Found on the Pacific Coast Trail, by Cheryl Strayed. Vintage Books, 2013.

INDEX

ABOUT THE AUTHOR

Sarah Hays Coomer is a self-proclaimed "diet-abolitionist." She is a certified personal trainer with the National Strength and Conditioning Association; a member of the American College of Sports Medicine; and a certified Nutrition and Wellness Consultant and Pre/Postnatal Fitness Specialist with the American Fitness Professionals Association. Sarah is a contributor to the *Nashville Scene* and writes a column for *The East Nashvillian* called "Simple Pleasures." She kind of likes to exercise, kind of not, and loves all things sugared, salted, fried, or dipped in dark chocolate. You can find her atwww.strengthoutsidein. com, on Twitter @strengthoutside, or Instagram @strengthoutsidein.